INTEGRATIVE COGNITIVE–AFFECTIVE THERAPY FOR BULIMIA NERVOSA

Integrative Cognitive–Affective Therapy for **Bulimia Nervosa**

A Treatment Manual

Stephen A. Wonderlich, Carol B. Peterson, and Tracey Leone Smith

with Marjorie H. Klein, James E. Mitchell, and Scott J. Crow

THE GUILFORD PRESS
New York   London

© 2015 The Guilford Press
A Division of Guilford Publications, Inc.
370 Seventh Avenue, Suite 1200, New York, NY 10001
www.guilford.com

Printed in the United States of America

This book is printed on acid-free paper.

Last digit is print number: 9   8   7   6   5   4   3   2   1

The authors have checked with sources believed to be reliable in their efforts to provide information that is complete and generally in accord with the standards of practice that are accepted at the time of publication. However, in view of the possibility of human error or changes in behavioral, mental health, or medical sciences, neither the authors, nor the editor and publisher, nor any other party who has been involved in the preparation or publication of this work warrants that the information contained herein is in every respect accurate or complete, and they are not responsible for any errors or omissions or the results obtained from the use of such information. Readers are encouraged to confirm the information contained in this book with other sources.

Library of Congress Cataloging-in-Publication Data

Wonderlich, Stephen.
   Integrative cognitive–affective therapy for bulimia nervosa : a treatment manual / by Stephen A. Wonderlich, Carol B. Peterson, and Tracey Leone Smith.
      pages cm
   Includes bibliographical references and index.
   ISBN 978-1-4625-2199-9 (paperback)
   1. Bulimia—Treatment—Handbooks, manuals, etc.   2. Cognitive therapy—Handbooks, manuals, etc.   I. Peterson, Carol B.   II. Smith, Tracey Leone, 1957–
   RC552.B84W66 2015
   616.85′2630651—dc23

2015014549

To our teachers, our patients,
and the individuals who participated in our studies

About the Authors

Stephen A. Wonderlich, PhD, the Chester Fritz Distinguished University Professor in the Department of Clinical Neuroscience at the University of North Dakota School of Medicine and Health Sciences and Director of Clinical Research at the Neuropsychiatric Research Institute. He is also Chairperson of the Eating Disorder Department at Sanford Health in Fargo, North Dakota. Dr. Wonderlich was president of the Academy for Eating Disorders in 1999–2000 and currently serves on several journal editorial boards. He is a recipient of the Academy for Eating Disorders Leadership Award in Research and the National Eating Disorders Association Price Family Award for Research Excellence. Dr. Wonderlich's research interests include the development of new treatments for individuals with eating disorders and identification of factors that either maintain or increase the risk for eating disorders. He publishes widely in the psychology and psychiatry literature and is the author or editor of six other books.

Carol B. Peterson, PhD, is Associate Professor in the Department of Psychiatry and Adjunct Assistant Professor in the Department of Psychology at the University of Minnesota. She is a Fellow of the Academy for Eating Disorders and a member of the editorial board of the *International Journal of Eating Disorders*. Dr. Peterson's research focuses on the assessment, diagnosis, and treatment of eating disorders, particularly psychotherapy treatment outcome studies. She also maintains a clinical practice and is Training Director at The Emily Program, an eating disorders treatment center.

Tracey Leone Smith, PhD, is Associate Professor in the Menninger Department of Psychiatry and Behavioral Sciences at Baylor College of Medicine in Houston. She serves as Psychotherapy Coordinator for the Department of Veterans Affairs (VA) in Mental Health Services in the VA Central Office. Her research has focused broadly on psychotherapy research, personality disorders, and the interpersonal processes that contribute to the etiology and treatment of mental health problems.

Marjorie H. Klein, PhD, is Professor of Psychiatry (Emeritus) in the Department of Psychiatry at the University of Wisconsin Medical School and in the Women's Studies Program at the University of Wisconsin. Her research has focused primarily on psychotherapy process and outcome research. Dr. Klein has developed methods for assessing patient experiential involvement and change in psychotherapy and measures for personality disorders and personality change. Other research has focused on the role of stress in family functioning and child development. Over the past 25 years, Dr. Klein has served on numerous National Institute of Mental Health Grant and Program Review Committees. She has published more than 100 journal articles and three books; given more than 130 presentations; and served on the editorial boards of seven journals, including *The Journal of Psychotherapy Practice and Research* and the *Journal of Personality Disorders*.

James E. Mitchell, MD, is the NRI/Lee A. Christoferson M.D. Professor and Chairman of the Department of Clinical Neuroscience at the University of North Dakota School of Medicine and Health Sciences. He is also the Chester Fritz Distinguished University Professor and serves as president and Scientific Director of the Neuropsychiatric Research Institute. Dr. Mitchell's research focuses on eating disorders, obesity, and bariatric surgery. He is past president of the Academy for Eating Disorders and the Eating Disorders Research Society and a recipient of the Academy for Eating Disorders Lifetime Achievement Award for Research in Eating Disorders, the National Eating Disorders Coalition Award for Research Leadership, and the Eating Disorders Research Society Research Award. Dr. Mitchell serves on the editorial boards of the *International Journal of Eating Disorders* and *Surgery for Obesity and Related Diseases*. He has written over 500 scientific articles and is author, coauthor, or editor of 18 other books.

Scott J. Crow, MD, is Professor of Psychiatry at the University of Minnesota and Director of Research at The Emily Program. He is also Program Director for the Midwest Regional Postdoctoral Training Program in Eating Disorders Research. Dr. Crow's research focuses on eating disorders and obesity. He is past president of the Academy for Eating Disorders and is Editor in Chief of *The Eating Disorders Review*. He has written over 200 scientific articles in the fields of eating disorders and obesity.

Acknowledgments

We are extremely grateful to a large number of people who have assisted us in the various stages of development of integrative cognitive–affective therapy (ICAT) for bulimia nervosa. Specifically, we would like to acknowledge our colleagues who contributed to the ecological momentary assessment studies that provided a foundation for the development of ICAT, as well as the individuals who contributed to the randomized controlled trial comparing ICAT to enhanced cognitive behavior therapy. These colleagues include Ross Crosby, PhD, Scott Engel, PhD, Joshua Smyth, PhD, Ray Miltenberger, PhD, Heather Simonich, MA, Daniel Le Grange, PhD, Jason Lavender, PhD, Li Cao, MS, Chad Lystad, MS, Nora Durkin, MA, Kelly Berg, PhD, Jessica McManus, MA, Aimee Arikian, PhD, Leah Jappe Hall, PhD, Annie Erickson, BA, Ron Erickson, MBA, Aimee Kurian, MS, Sara Anderson, BS, Desiree Cabinte, MS, and Timothy Baardseth, MS.

We would also like to express our gratitude to the psychologists who served as clinicians in the controlled trial of ICAT for bulimia nervosa: Tricia Myers, PhD, Lorraine Swan-Kremeier, PsyD, and Kathryn Miller, PhD. We would also like to acknowledge the support we received from the National Institute of Mental Health (MH077571), which made the development of ICAT possible, and particularly Dr. Mark Chavez, whose support of the work was essential. Additionally, our home institutions (University of North Dakota School of Medicine and Health Sciences/ Neuropsychiatric Research Institute, University of Minnesota, University of Wisconsin, Sanford Health, and Baylor College of Medicine) all provided various types of support that allowed us to conduct our research and clinical work.

Last, several people assisted us in translating the results of our scientific studies into what we believe is a clinically relevant and useful book outlining the essentials of ICAT. In particular, we would like to thank Vonnie Sandland for her endless clerical support and Dr. Jo Ellison, who, during her postdoctoral fellowship, took on a part-time project as a copy editor of earlier drafts of the manuscript. Additionally, we appreciate the thoughtful and astute contributions of Jim Nageotte and Jane Keislar at The Guilford Press.

Contents

PART III. ICAT-BN PATIENT HANDOUTS
AND SKILL CARDS

INTEGRATIVE COGNITIVE–AFFECTIVE THERAPY FOR BULIMIA NERVOSA

Introduction

WHAT IS ICAT-BN?

This book describes integrative cognitive–affective therapy for bulimia nervosa (ICAT-BN) and includes descriptions of its structure, process, and techniques. ICAT-BN is a short-term, structured treatment that is designed to be conducted over a minimum of 21 sessions, each approximately 45–50 minutes in length. Although ICAT-BN shares several features with other treatments for bulimia nervosa (BN), it also includes several unique concepts and interventions. Consistent with other evidence-based treatments, this manual provides clinicians with information regarding treatment content, structure, and format based on a protocol that has been demonstrated to be efficacious in a randomized controlled trial (Wonderlich et al., 2014). ICAT-BN also includes a number of patient-oriented handouts and treatment supplements such as skill cards that highlight the ICAT-BN skills. ICAT-BN is based on models of conditioning and learning as applied to eating disorder behavior, which guide many of the interventions throughout the treatment. It retains various elements of traditional behavioral therapy including self-monitoring, planned meals, and direct efforts to modify behaviors.

However, ICAT-BN is more specifically influenced by an underlying model of psychopathology, and the treatment is based on a momentary model of the maintenance of BN behavior. The momentary nature of the underlying model is clearly detectable and emphasized throughout ICAT-BN. ICAT-BN is also an emotion-focused treatment that emphasizes the functional relationship between emotional states and bulimic behavior. Although ICAT-BN highlights the development of emotion-regulation skills, it is not simply a didactic intervention. Rather, it relies on a collaborative psychotherapeutic relationship in which the patient and the clinician are clearly working together to set goals and address the relationship between emotional experience and bulimic behavior.

HOW THIS BOOK IS ORGANIZED

This book is organized into three main sections. Part I (Chapters 1–4) is an introduction to BN and ICAT-BN. Chapter 1 presents an overview of BN, its diagnosis, medical complications, and treatments. Chapter 2 describes the models of BN onset and maintenance that underlie the treatment presented in this book. Chapter 3 describes ICAT's emotion focus, structure, goals, and strategies. Chapter 4 describes the core skills taught to patients and the essential role of the therapeutic relationship. Part II (Chapters 5–8) details how to implement ICAT. Each of the four chapters in Part II describes a phase of the treatment. Part III of the book contains all of ICAT's patient-oriented handouts and treatment supplements, such as skill cards for the ICAT-BN skills. Permission is granted to individual book purchasers to photocopy these materials and to download and print them from the publisher's website for their personal use with patients. Please see the copyright page for details.

THE EVOLUTION OF ICAT-BN

In 1996, researchers from the University of North Dakota/Neuropsychiatric Research Institute (Wonderlich, Mitchell, Crosby, and their colleagues) and the University of Minnesota, Department of Psychiatry (Peterson, Crow, Mussell, and their colleagues) began a series of meetings that extended over several years. Our goal was to discuss a variety of research topics related to eating disorders and obesity, including the idea of developing innovative treatment models. The clinicians and scientists involved in these meetings had a lengthy history of collaborative research on a variety of topics related to eating disorders, including empirical studies of treatment outcome. The discussions in these meetings were wide ranging and covered issues related to diagnostics, etiology, comorbidity, and, most consistently, innovative ideas about treatment. For example, we formulated ideas that led to successful treatment trials involving telemedicine-based delivery of BN treatment, self-help treatment for binge-eating disorder, and a stepped-care model for BN treatment. During this time we were also developing a platform to conduct ecological momentary assessment (EMA) studies, in which participants would carry a "personal digital assistant" and provide reports on their eating disorder behaviors and experiences in real time in the natural environment. The one topic that proved somewhat elusive was our desire to develop an innovative theoretical model of the psychopathology of BN, and a treatment based on that model. Over the next 10 years we considered various constructs in the model, completed descriptive psychopathology studies, wrote drafts of treatment manuals, and conducted pilot studies of new intervention approaches, which ultimately led to ICAT-BN.

Based on our reading of the literature as well as our clinical experience, we began to consider individual difference constructs like self-evaluation and interpersonal relationship factors in the onset and/or maintenance of bulimic behavior. We were also interested in the role of emotional variables and the possible functional relationship that bulimic behaviors may have with such affective processes, which was a primary focus of our EMA studies. At the same time, we did not want to lose track of what we thought were important scientific and clinical findings that had already emerged in the eating disorder literature. For example, we recognized the importance of dietary restraint and food restriction to bulimic behavior and the value of self-monitoring and direct behavioral strategies to modify eating behavior, particularly in the early phases of treatment for BN.

As we progressed toward a more integrative approach to treatment, we were fortunate to engage Marjorie (Marj) Klein, from the University of Wisconsin–Madison, to join us in our collaboration. Marj had connections to the North Dakota group and was serving as a consultant on their EMA study of bulimic behavior. Marj was not well acquainted with BN or eating disorders but had considerable expertise in psychotherapy research, dating back to her work with Carl Rogers, as well as her well-known work in personality disorders. Her expertise provided us with the integrative breadth we needed to move toward a broader model of BN. At about this point, around the year 2000, we began to develop drafts of a manual for a treatment of BN based on our evolving model of bulimic behavior. Conversations with another Wisconsin colleague (Tim Strauman) led us to the idea that disparities between one's perception of one's actual self and one's comparative evaluative standards for the actual self (i.e., self-discrepancy) could elicit significant levels of negative affect, an idea we thought was relevant to BN. We conducted a series of different types of descriptive, correlational studies examining the relationship between self-discrepancy and bulimic behavior and repeatedly found significant associations, which supported our idea that this construct had potential clinical significance. We began to ponder how self-discrepancy, negative affect, interpersonal relationships, and bulimic behavior might be related. These considerations led to the first version of our manual, entitled *Integrative Cognitive Therapy (ICT)*. Initially, we treated nine BN cases in Fargo, North Dakota, and Minneapolis, Minnesota, with ICT. Most of these cases helped us to learn how patients thought about ideas like self-discrepancy and its link to emotion. This connection seemed compelling, but the link between emotion and bulimic behavior was more complicated. Individuals in treatment often thought they binge ate or purged because they were "upset," but we could not determine if emotion was better viewed as a true antecedent of bulimic behavior or a post hoc explanation that did not really predict BN behavior.

Importantly, at the time that this treatment was evolving, several of us from Fargo (Wonderlich, Crosby, Engel, and Mitchell) were progressing in our EMA studies with individuals with BN. In retrospect, it seems somewhat coincidental that our EMA studies were focused on momentary relationships between emotional states and bulimic behavior while we were simultaneously discussing similar emotional processes in our treatment protocol for BN. With EMA we were able to demonstrate that negative emotional states seemed to be reliable predictors of episodes of bulimic behavior over relatively short intervals (i.e., minutes to hours). Yet, the relevance of these emotion-related findings for treatment was not clear to any of us. We began to recognize that if this trajectory of negative emotional states leading to bulimic behavior could be influenced, we might be able to change the likelihood of bulimic episodes. As a result, our treatment development process took a decided turn toward the role of emotion in treatment. We read the works of clinical scientists who included emotion-related variables in their treatments (e.g., Barlow, Hayes, Greenberg, Benjamin, Mennin, and Linehan) and emotion-regulation theorists (e.g., Gratz, Gross, Campos, and Thompson), all of which helped clarify our thinking about emotional experience in BN. As a result, ICT became significantly more "affective," and this resulted in a small but significant change in the title of the treatment: integrative cognitive therapy (i.e., ICT) became integrative cognitive–affective therapy (ICAT).

In 2003, we continued to modify our treatment manual, and in our efforts to do so added another collaborator, Tracey Smith, who was also at the University of Wisconsin. Tracey had experience working in the area of treatment manual development and psychotherapy adherence; she was also familiar with treatments informed by interpersonal and emotional processes. After another year of considerable modifications to our original manual, another pilot study was conducted in Fargo, Minneapolis, and Madison. Eight more individuals with BN were treated, and we remained cautiously optimistic about the potential efficacy of our treatment. As our thinking and clinical technique continued to evolve, we began to consider opportunities to conduct larger studies, which led to an application to the National Institute of Mental Health to conduct a treatment development project, which was ultimately funded in 2006. This grant provided an opportunity to further refine our manuals and then conduct a randomized controlled trial comparing ICAT-BN to the most well-established, evidence-based treatment for BN, enhanced cognitive behavior therapy (CBT-E; Fairburn, 2008). This study, conducted in Fargo and Minneapolis with the University of Wisconsin serving as the therapy adherence center, took place between 2007 and 2011. Eighty individuals with BN were randomized to either CBT-E or ICAT for a 21-session treatment conducted over 17 weeks. Four doctoral-level psychologists (Carol Peterson, Kathryn Miller, Tricia Myers, and Lorraine Swan-Kremeier), who had all served as clinicians delivering CBT in previous randomized controlled trials for BN, were trained in both CBT-E and ICAT-BN. Chris Fairburn's colleague Zafra Cooper provided periodic consultation on the implementation of CBT-E. Two of us (S. A. W. and C. B. P.) provided ICAT-BN supervision. The results of the study (Wonderlich et al., 2014) suggested that each treatment was reliably administered, and each treatment displayed significant ability to reduce key features of BN and associated psychopathology (e.g., depression, anxiety). There were no differences between the two treatments at outcome at the end of treatment or at 4-month follow-up. Based on the reasonable performance of ICAT-BN in this trial, along with our successful piloting of the treatment, we elected to write this treatment manual.

One of the most striking features of ICAT-BN to emerge over the last several years has been an appreciation of the clinical relevance of the momentary relationship of emotions and BN behavior that we observed in our EMA studies. Although we had originally considered emotional states to be important to the onset and maintenance of BN behavior, we had not carefully considered the temporal framework of this relationship. Cross-sectional research designs and longitudinal studies with several months between assessment intervals suggested that emotion was somehow relevant to BN, but the nature of this association eluded us. We were inclined to consider the emotion variable as a trait-like construct on which individuals with BN had deficits. This assumption led us to think about ways to educate individuals with BN about emotional states and how to generally prepare them to manage emotions effectively, almost like a basic "101" course in emotional intelligence. What we failed to appreciate at that time was that emotional states appear to be significantly and reliably changing in relatively brief periods of time before the occurrence of bulimic episodes, an observation that was made clear in our EMA data. In the moments and hours before binge eating and purge behavior occurred, negative affect was rising and positive affect was decreasing. This finding forced us to consider more rigorously the time frame for the relationship between emotional states and bulimic behavior. Our EMA data differed from previous studies using cross-sectional research designs or a time-lagged association design in which emotions and bulimic behaviors were often separated by months or even years. This helped us to shift our focus from helping patients with BN improve their general emotional functioning to assisting them in identifying and managing emotions in the moments before a bulimic episode. As a result, ICAT-BN became a treatment that attempted to modify momentary variables surrounding BN behavior. The treatment moved in the direction of a much more situationally specific context in which particular interpersonal or intrapersonal antecedents were thought to trigger emotional changes, which in turn precipitated BN behavior at a particular time. This focus meant encouraging patients to more closely monitor episodes of BN behavior, situations that preceded the behavior, and the emotions that followed. Treatment became more focused on emotionally laden situations and the decisions to engage in binge eating, purging, and the various behaviors in BN. Also, we began to discuss with our patients what role or function the BN behavior may have played for them at the time it occurred, which seemed to facilitate a different perspective on the behavior. Moreover, the emphasis on emotions seemed to intensify the clinical sessions. We strove to find emotionally meaningful moments and their connection to BN behavior. Identifying situations that elicited strong emotion became important, as did the experience of the emotion to the patient, both retrospectively as they recalled it and in the session itself. The combination of an emotion focus and the momentary time frame seemed to bring an intensity and relevance to ICAT-BN that the clinicians perceived as different from other BN treatments they had delivered.

Another aspect of ICAT-BN that has continued to evolve over time, particularly in the last few years, has been our understanding of impulsivity and rash decision making in the treatment. From its inception, ICAT-BN has been oriented toward the idea that individuals with BN have difficulty inhibiting impulsive behaviors. Like many researchers, we have been examining the relationship between impulsivity and BN over the last 25–30 years. However, a particular form of impulsivity, negative urgency, had a significant impact on our recent thinking about treatment. Negative urgency refers to a propensity to act rashly in the face of negative emotional experience. The concept of negative urgency, which integrates emotion regulation and impulsive action, was an excellent fit for ICAT-BN. It helped us to identify an additional element that needed to be included in the intervention, namely, helping individuals with BN develop some degree of control and restraint over their impulsive actions, particularly their eating disorder symptoms. Consequently, in addition to facilitating a greater awareness of situational and emotional cues for bulimic behavior, we also help our patients develop adaptive coping behavior that they can use to inhibit such impulsive action.

To summarize, ICAT-BN has evolved over nearly 20 years of development and currently offers several key interventional elements to (1) improve an individual's awareness and tolerance of emotional experience; (2) formulate a well-structured plan to modify eating behavior; (3) develop skills to reduce the likelihood of rash, impulsive behaviors (particularly in the context of negative emotion); and (4) identify cues for emotional experience and modify the source of increased negative emotions or decreased positive emotions in the individual's life.

Part I

CONCEPTUAL AND CLINICAL
FOUNDATIONS OF ICAT-BN

Chapter 1

An Overview of Bulimia Nervosa
Diagnosis, Complications, and Treatment

Although isolated case reports and series have appeared in the literature for a number of decades, the syndrome of BN was first described by Russell in a 1979 paper, in which the condition was conceptualized as a variant of anorexia nervosa (AN). Over the last 35 years, BN has been recognized as a distinct and significant psychiatric disorder. It was first included in DSM III-R (American Psychiatric Association [APA], 1987). The diagnostic criteria were revised in DSM-IV (APA, 1994) and in DSM-5 (APA, 2013). Prevalence estimates indicate that 1–3.5% of females between the ages of 15 and 30 have met DSM-IV diagnostic criteria (Hoek & van Hoeken, 2003; Hudson, Hiripi, Pope, & Kessler, 2007). Among males, the prevalence is less and estimated to be about 0.5% (Hudson et al., 2007). However, epidemiological studies suggest a larger percentage of both males and females have bulimic symptoms without meeting all of the clinical diagnostic criteria (Hoek & van Hoeken, 2003). This is important due to the growing recognition that subclinical forms of BN do not differ significantly from full-syndrome BN in a variety of comparisons across social and medical criteria (Thomas, Vartanian, & Brownell, 2009). Consistent with the growing recognition of the severity of subclinical BN, the DSM-5 diagnostic criteria reduced the frequency of binge–purge behavior from twice to once per week (see Table 1.1). This relatively small change in the frequency of symptoms was intended to reduce the number of individuals who did not meet DSM-IV diagnostic criteria for BN and were classified as eating disorder not otherwise specified (EDNOS).

BN usually begins in late adolescence or young adulthood, with most studies reporting a mean age of onset around 19 to 20 years (Hudson et al., 2007). Many patients are symptomatic for several years before seeking treatment, and it is often

TABLE 1.1. DSM-5 Diagnostic Criteria for BN

A. Recurrent episodes of binge eating. An episode of binge eating is characterized by both of the following:

    1. Eating, in a discrete period of time (e.g., within any 2-hour period), an amount of food that is definitely larger than what most individuals would eat in a similar period of time under similar circumstances.

    2. A sense of lack of control over eating during the episode (e.g., a feeling that one cannot stop eating or control what or how much one is eating).

B. Recurrent inappropriate compensatory behaviors in order to prevent weight gain, such as self-induced vomiting; misuse of laxatives, diuretics, or other medications; fasting; or excessive exercise.

C. The binge eating and inappropriate compensatory behaviors both occur, on average, at least once a week for 3 months.

D. Self-evaluation is unduly influenced by body shape and weight.

E. The disturbance does not occur exclusively during episodes of anorexia nervosa.

Note. Reprinted with permission from the *Diagnostic and Statistical Manual of Mental Disorders, Fifth Edition.* Copyright 2013 by the American Psychiatric Association. All rights reserved.

the consequences of the disorder, rather than the eating behaviors per se, that eventually lead them to seek treatment (e.g., medical problems, depression, or psychosocial impairment). Although the diagnostic criteria require only that patients with BN binge-eat and use compensatory behaviors at least once a week for 3 months, typical patients with BN binge-eat once or twice a day, and sometimes more frequently (Mitchell, Hatsukami, Eckert, & Pyle, 1985a; Powers, 1996). There is a great deal of variability in what constitutes binge-eating behavior, but usually large amounts of food are consumed, often in excess of 1,000 calories or more (Mitchell, Crow, Peterson, Wonderlich, & Crosby, 1998; Walsh, Kissileff, & Hadigan, 1989). Furthermore, following binge-eating episodes many patients engage in self-induced vomiting, which is the most common compensatory behavior. Most patients with BN (i.e., 88%; Mitchell et al., 1985a) begin to self-induce vomiting by using some form of mechanical manipulation, such as inserting their hand or a toothbrush into their throat, while many eventually learn to vomit reflexively over the years and do not require mechanical stimulation to vomit by the time they seek treatment. It is important to note, however, that vomiting may occur in the absence of binge eating.

Although binge eating and self-induced vomiting are the most common features of BN, a number of other problematic compensatory and associated behaviors can co-occur as summarized in Table 1.2 (Mitchell, Hatsukami, Pyle, & Eckert, 1988). These include misuse of laxatives (approximately 60% at least intermittently), over-the-counter diet pills (at least 50% intermittently), diuretics (about 15%, usually

TABLE 1.2. Other Common Features of BN

Cognitive/emotional
- Depression
- Irritability
- Problems concentrating
- Anxiety

Financial/social
- Financial problems, including loss of savings, borrowing from friends, and debt
- Feeling socially isolated from family and friends, in part because of the secretive nature of bulimic symptoms
- Work and school may be problematic with lack of advancement and poor attendance
- Sometimes people develop legal problems for writing bad checks or shoplifting

Medical
- Electrolyte abnormalities
- Menstrual irregularity
- Salivary gland swelling
- Tooth enamel erosion
- Rarely gastric dilatation and esophageal rupture

Behavioral
Often as a consequence of the disorder:
- Dishonesty
- Stealing
- Misuse alcohol or drugs
- Struggle with relationships

over-the-counter diuretics, but some abuse of prescription diuretics), rumination (as high as 33% of subjects in some studies), and, in the past when it was widely available, ipecac (experimentation by approximately 12% of patients with BN, with regular usage in 2–3%) (Mitchell, Hatsukami, Pyle, & Eckert, 1986). Other compensatory behaviors are seen less frequently, including misuse of saunas, enemas, thyroid medication, and insulin (among individuals with diabetes) (Mitchell, Pyle, & Eckert, 1991a; Mitchell, Pyle, & Hatsukami, 1991b). Patients with BN frequently have significant social impairment, similar to that of women undergoing treatment for substance abuse (Holderness, Brooks-Gunn, & Warren, 1994) and reporting long-term social impairment over the course of the disorder (Keel, Mitchell, Miller, Davis, & Crow, 1999).

Patients with BN frequently experience other comorbid psychiatric conditions (Wonderlich & Mitchell, 1997), and although the exact relationship between BN and these other conditions is not always clear, psychiatric comorbidity is so common that it becomes a major influence in terms of treatment planning (Fichter & Quadflieg, 2004; Milos, Spindler, Ruggiero, Klaghofer, & Schnyder, 2002). One of the most common comorbidities is major depressive disorder. Approximately 80% of patients with BN will have a lifetime history of depression, and 50% will have active depression when seen for evaluation (Herzog, Keller, Sachs, Yeh, & Lavori, 1992). Anxiety disorders are also commonly observed, particularly social phobia and panic disorder (Hudson et al., 2007; Laessle, Wittchen, Fichter, & Pirke, 1989), as well as substance use problems involving alcohol and drugs (Herzog et al., 1992). In some studies, as many as 20–25% of individuals with BN have significant alcohol or other drug use disorders (Bulik, Sullivan, & Epstein, 1992). Personality disorders, particularly DSM-IV Cluster B and C disturbances, are also common in women with BN and are of particular relevance to treatment (Cassin & von Ranson, 2005). The presence of a Cluster B personality disorder has been shown to be a negative outcome predictor for some treatments (Rossiter, Agras, Telch, & Schneider, 1993), although this finding has been inconsistently demonstrated (Grilo et al., 2007).

The course of BN is highly variable, with some patients experiencing a nonremitting, chronic course and others experiencing waxing and waning of symptoms over time (Keel et al., 1999), or migrating to another eating disorder diagnosis (Fairburn & Harrison, 2003). Long-term follow-up studies suggest that many patients do recover eventually without treatment, but a subgroup continue a chronic course and are still symptomatic at long-term follow-up (Keel & Mitchell, 1997; Keel et al., 1999). Studies of relapse suggest that patients who are abstinent from bulimic symptoms at the end of treatment and are able to maintain their abstinence for a period of 6 months are less likely to relapse subsequently (Mitchell, Davis & Goff, 1985b). Furthermore, abstinence from bulimic symptoms at the end of treatment is an important predictor of 6-month and long-term outcome (Maddocks, Kaplan, Woodside, Langdon, & Prian, 1992).

MEDICAL COMPLICATIONS

Although medical morbidity is fairly common in BN, mortality is generally considered relatively rare in contrast to the significant mortality rate associated with AN (Berkman, Lohr, & Bulik, 2007; Hoek, 2006). However, a recent study indicates that mortality rates for BN, as well as EDNOS, which may include subclinical forms of BN, are higher than was once assumed (Crow et al., 2009). The most frequent medical complications of BN are nonspecific physical complaints including weakness, fatigue, and dizziness. Comorbid depression may confound the accurate assessment of medical complaints.

The most frequent system-related physical abnormalities in BN are fluid/electrolyte abnormalities (Mitchell & Crow, 2006) including hypochloremia (decreased serum chloride), metabolic alkalosis (increased serum bicarbonate), and hypokalemia (decreased serum potassium). These conditions develop because of the loss of hydrogen in the vomitus and fluid contraction, with the subsequent shift of potassium into the cells and loss of potassium through the urine. Hypokalemia is particularly problematic because it raises concerns about cardiac conduction abnormalities. Patients who abuse laxatives or diuretics can have metabolic acidosis, at least transiently (decreased serum bicarbonate). Approximately 50% of patients with BN will show abnormalities on measures of serum electrolytes (Greenfeld, Mickley, Quinlan, & Roloff, 1995).

Another common medical complication of BN is loss of dental enamel associated with vomiting (Simmons, Grayden, & Mitchell, 1986). These dental changes are usually greatest on the lingual or posterior surface of the upper teeth, where the vomitus makes contact as it is projected from the throat during the act of vomiting. Typically, enamel erosion occurs around the amalgams or fillings, which are resistant to the acid and end up floating like "islands" above the surface of the tooth with the enamel washed out around them.

An extremely serious but rare complication of BN is gastric dilatation, in which the patient is unable to vomit and has continued expansion of the stomach secondary to fluid release into the lumen of the stomach following a binge-eating episode (Bravender & Story, 2007; Carney & Andersen, 1996). This condition requires surgical consultation and may require surgical decompression. Gastric rupture can lead to death. Cases of esophageal rupture (with vomiting), a condition that is also potentially fatal, have been reported (Abdu, Garritano, & Culver, 1987).

Many patients with BN will complain of irregular menses, although amenorrhea is less common than in AN (Crow, Agras, Halmi, Mitchell, & Kraemer, 2002). Neuroendocrine hypothalamic–pituitary–ovarian hormones are frequently dysregulated as part of the disorder. There is also evidence of abnormalities in the regulation of other hormonal systems, including prolactin and cortisol (Ferrari et al., 1997; Birketvedt et al., 2006), although the clinical significance of these changes is less clear.

Overall, the main sources of clinical concern in BN are fluid and electrolyte abnormalities, dental enamel erosion, and the risk of rare and dangerous complications such as gastric dilatation and esophageal rupture. For these reasons, individuals with bulimic symptoms need to be monitored to ensure medical stability.

TREATMENTS FOR BN

Since the original description of BN in 1979 (Russell, 1979), an impressive literature has developed on the treatment of this disorder. It has mainly followed two paths: pharmacotherapy approaches that have relied primarily on antidepressant drugs and psychotherapy approaches that have focused primarily on cognitive-behavioral techniques. The available treatment studies using antidepressant medications show quite clearly that many of the available drugs suppress binge eating and vomiting and can improve mood in patients with BN, although most patients are not free of symptoms at the end of drug treatment (Jimerson, Wolfe, Brotman, & Metzger, 1996). Tricyclic antidepressants (e.g., imipramine, desipramine) were the first antidepressants shown to be helpful in the treatment of BN. Serotonin reuptake inhibitors also work for some individuals, and now because of their safety are typically used instead of the tricyclics. The drug that has been studied most extensively is fluoxetine hydrochloride (Prozac), which remains the only drug approved by the Food and Drug Administration (FDA) for the treatment of BN in the United States. It is often given at a dose of 60 milligrams a day, in contrast to the 20-milligram dose often effective for the treatment of depression (Goldstein, Wilson, Thompson, Potvin, & Rampay, 1995). Other experimental drug treatments are often used to treat bulimic symptoms as well as the depression and anxiety that often occur with BN. Pharmacological interventions, when used alone, rarely produce enduring remissions, and many patients become more symptomatic once they are removed from the medication (Fairburn, 2008). Combinations of treatment may also be effective. Combining drug treatment (e.g., fluoxetine) with psychological therapies may be better than either treatment alone for some patients, but psychological therapy (e.g., cognitive-behavioral therapy [CBT]) without medication has been found to be as effective as psychological treatment with medication (Wilson, Grilo, & Vitousek, 2007). Although people with BN are usually treated in outpatient settings, some need to be treated in hospital-based programs.

CBT was developed by Beck (1967, 1976, 1987) for the treatment of depression and has been adapted for the treatment of BN (Fairburn, 2008; Fairburn, Marcus, & Wilson, 1993b). Administered in both individual and group formats, CBT has been shown to be the preferred manual-based psychotherapy approach to treatment of BN (Wonderlich, de Zwaan, Mitchell, Peterson, & Crow, 2003). It has been shown to work as well as, or better, than all control treatments, and clearly is superior to waiting-list controls, minimal intervention controls, or nonspecific supportive interventions (Fairburn et al., 1993b). Interpersonal therapy (IPT; Fairburn, 1997), another psychotherapy approach developed for the treatment of depression that has been adapted for BN, focuses on addressing current interpersonal relationship problems that are hypothesized to maintain the eating disorder symptoms. Several empirical comparisons have shown that IPT is comparable to CBT in terms of improvements in bulimic symptoms, although IPT appears to act more slowly than CBT (Fairburn et al., 1993a, 1995; Agras, Walsh, Fairburn, Wilson, & Kraemer, 1999).

Currently, CBT (e.g., Agras et al., 1992; Fairburn et al., 1993b; Fairburn, 2008; Mitchell et al., 1990) is the most widely tested and effective form of treatment for BN. In the National Institute for Clinical Excellence (now the National Institute for Health and Care Excellence [NICE]) Guidelines (2004), CBT for BN was given an A grade as an evidence-based treatment (IPT was given a B grade for the treatment of BN). However, many patients, even if improved, remain symptomatic after CBT; additional CBT limitations include significant dropout and relapse rates (Mitchell, Hoberman, Peterson, Mussell, & Pyle, 1996).

A recently developed version of CBT, CBT-E (Fairburn, 2008), which is intended to treat a full range of eating disorders, has received considerable clinical and scientific attention. CBT-E may be administered in either a focused or a broad clinical format. The focused approach resembles traditional CBT for BN, while the broad approach includes interventions that target a greater range of clinical constructs, such as clinical perfectionism, interpersonal problems, or core low self-esteem. In a randomized controlled trial involving 154 patients with eating disorders, many of whom had BN, over half of the participants receiving CBT-E showed what was deemed to be a clinically significant response based on the Eating Disorder Examination; furthermore, this treatment effect did not differ by eating disorder diagnosis. In a recent review, Fairburn and colleagues commented that it would appear as though CBT-E is more effective than traditional CBT (Murphy, Straebler, Cooper, & Fairburn, 2010).

Increasing evidence also suggests that self-help interventions, which involve the use of a treatment manual and often some form of supportive clinical assistance in applying the intervention, can also be useful in the treatment of BN (Wilson & Zandberg, 2012). In particular, guided self-help, which includes a limited number of supportive face-to-face sessions with a provider, has been shown to be effective in the treatment of BN. In one large trial comparing guided self-help to face-to-face CBT for BN, there were no significant differences in remission rates, and the authors concluded that guided self-help may be considered an effective first-line treatment for BN (Mitchell et al., 2011).

There is also a small amount of evidence to suggest that a modified version of dialectical behavior therapy (DBT) for eating disorders may be effective in the treatment of BN. This DBT-based treatment is generally considered appropriate for individuals with binge-eating problems and has been tested for individuals with binge-eating disorder as well as BN. In one randomized controlled trial of DBT for BN (Safer, Telch, & Agras, 2001), participants received either DBT skills training or a wait-list control condition. At the end of treatment, over one quarter of the BN participants receiving DBT reported abstinence from binge eating and purging, while none of the wait-list participants reported abstinence. These findings offer preliminary data to suggest that skill-oriented affect regulation treatment may be useful in the treatment of BN.

Finally, ICAT-BN was recently compared to CBT-E in a randomized controlled trial. Eighty participants meeting diagnostic criteria for full-syndrome or subclinical BN received either ICAT-BN or CBT-E over 21 sessions of treatment. Both treatments were associated with significant improvement in bulimic symptoms as well as all other outcome measures, and there were no significant differences observed between the two treatment conditions at end of treatment or at 4-month follow-up. Intent-to-treat abstinence rates for ICAT-BN were 37.5% at the end of treatment, compared to 22.5% for CBT-E. In general, both treatments maintained these gains at the follow-up assessment. This study supports the efficacy of ICAT-BN as well as the possibility that it is comparable to CBT-E, an established treatment for BN.

LIVING WITH BN: THE STORIES BEHIND THE DATA

Important as scientific data and diagnostic criteria are in understanding the phenomena of BN, they do not adequately portray the experience of people suffering from this disorder. The following case examples[1] illustrate the wide variety of individuals who suffer from BN, the variability of the disorder, and the human toll of bulimic symptoms.

Case Example: Sydney

Sydney is an 18-year-old college student who started binge eating and vomiting at age 15. As a child, Sydney was shy and anxious, and her family still teases her about her separation anxiety when she attended elementary school. She laughs when they tease her, but recalling that time is still very painful for her. Sydney also remembers worrying about disappointing her family and teachers and striving to be "perfect" at school, sports, and activities. A competitive tennis player, Sydney was ranked in the upper tier of players in her state starting at age 10. She reports that she was always so nervous about matches that she was unable to sleep the night before as she worried about mistakes that she might make. A straight-A student as well as an accomplished tennis player, Sydney had a few close friends but spent the majority of her time outside of school traveling to matches with her mother and coach. She remembers that her eating disorder started at age 14 when she began menstruating and her coach criticized her for gaining weight. Ashamed, and fearing that puberty and the subsequent changes in her body weight would negatively impact her skills as a tennis player, Sydney began to increase her workouts off the court and became more focused on eating "healthy." She read books and online sources about sports nutrition and calculated calories and macronutrients in an attempt to lose weight.

At first, she was exhilarated by her weight loss, especially when she was praised by her coach for her self-discipline. As a result, she increased her workout frequency and intensity and spent less time socializing with her friends. After 6 months of this eating and exercise regimen, however, Sydney found herself more irritable and

---

[1]Cases reflect compilations of information from different individuals with identifying information deleted.

craving the foods that she restricted herself from eating. Criticizing herself for such "weakness," she resisted these urges until one afternoon, soon after she turned 15. In a high-profile tennis tournament, she lost to an opponent with a lower ranking. If that was not distressing enough, the loss was followed by Sydney's coach and mother expressing deep disappointment in her performance. Sydney went home after the tournament and cried in her room. Alone without anyone else in the house, she went downstairs and began eating foods that she had not allowed herself to eat in months, including desserts and snack food. Once she started, she could not stop herself. Finally, too full to continue, she looked at the empty wrappers in the kitchen, felt a sense of panic at the imminent weight gain that would result from having eaten so much food, and ran to the bathroom to self-induce vomiting. Relieved, she consoled herself by promising to never binge-eat and purge again. Three days later, however, she had another bulimic episode after she received a B minus on a math quiz. Within a month, she was binge eating and vomiting at least 4 days a week. In addition to the bulimic episodes, Sydney noticed that she was completely preoccupied with eating: when she would eat, what she had eaten, whether she would gain weight, and where she could purge. She found herself feeling tearful, irritable, and withdrawn from her friends, whom she believed she could not confide in for fear that they would criticize her. Sydney also noticed that she felt weak and dizzy as well as suffering from frequent stomach pain. Although she continued to receive high grades, her tennis skills suffered greatly, and by the age of 16, she was no longer ranked within the state. Sydney abandoned plans to attend college on an athletic scholarship, much to her family's disappointment. Nevertheless when she arrived at college, she looked forward to a "fresh start" with new friends, an academically rigorous curriculum, and, she hoped, freedom from her bulimic symptoms. For the first 3 weeks of school, she was able to resist binge eating and purging. However, prior to her first midterm exam, her bulimic pattern resumed, and when she sought treatment a month later, she was binge eating and purging daily.

Case Example: Ethan

Now age 25, Ethan remembers stealing boxes of sugar to eat in his room when he was only 5 years old. Secretly binge eating throughout childhood, Ethan was often teased about being overweight. He remembers that eating was soothing and comforting to him. He also remembers the intense pleasure that eating alone in his room would provide him. However, Ethan also recalls the shame that he felt when his family complained about food missing from the kitchen. The youngest of five children, he often felt lonely when the rest of his family was focused on the needs of his brothers and sisters. Nonetheless, he had a number of friends and was involved in many extracurricular activities, including theater and choir. Throughout high school and college, Ethan would alternate between month-long periods of binge eating and times when he would exercise daily and restrict how much he ate. Ethan had heard of BN but could not imagine making himself throw up until he was 21 and offered a role as an actor in a local community theater production. Concerned about "looking fat" on stage, Ethan found that he was unable to follow any of the diets that he had tried in the past. One day, in desperation, he tried self-induced vomiting after eating a large pizza. Although he was fearful that the experience might be disgusting, he was surprised to find that he was both relieved to be free of worry about weight gain and emotionally calmed by the act of binge eating and vomiting. After that first episode, Ethan would find himself binge eating and purging every time he felt badly about himself, overwhelmed by demands at school or lonely. Somewhat reluctantly, given his reliance on his bulimic symptoms to help regulate his mood and weight, Ethan decided to seek treatment because he feared the medical and emotional consequences of his bulimic symptoms.

Case Example: Cassidy

Cassidy was in and out of mental health treatments for a variety of psychological problems during her adolescence. As a young adult Cassidy describes her adolescence as "wild" and acknowledges using a variety of drugs, engaging in promiscuous sex, and having bulimic episodes intermittently. Having experienced ongoing sexual abuse by an uncle when she was young, Cassidy was seen by a number of counselors and therapists during childhood when a neighbor discovered the abuse and reported it to the authorities. Raised by a single mother who "hated" Cassidy's birth father (whom Cassidy has never met), Cassidy remembers moving frequently while she was growing up but finding that she could "fit in" regardless of the school she attended because she would identify "the partiers" at school, who would always welcome her. She started drinking alcohol daily at age 13 and using drugs, including daily marijuana and painkillers, at age 15. She remembers that her first purging episode occurred at age 16 because she "felt fat" and tried vomiting on a whim. She also reports having used laxatives and diuretics as well as vomiting in an attempt to control her weight. Cassidy says that since adolescence she has always been bulimic, substance dependent, or both (although more typically in an alternating pattern). She attended drug and alcohol treatment four times, starting at age 17, but never told anyone in these treatment centers that she had bulimic symptoms. In fact, she remembers binge eating and purging throughout all of her drug and alcohol treatments. Cassidy has volatile relationships with her family members and friends, as well as with her boyfriends. She describes feeling like love is a "drug" for her when she meets someone new and starts dating him; however, within a month, she becomes bored and ends the relationship. In spite of her chaotic lifestyle, Cassidy is a skilled salesperson and, other than when she was in rehab, has worked successfully in a series of sales jobs around the country. Uncertain about whether she should get treatment for her eating disorder, Cassidy considers her main priority to be her sobriety, which she has maintained for the past 2 years. However, she has noticed that her bulimic symptoms have gotten worse in the context of her sobriety and increased work travel. She is also concerned about finances because she spends so much of her income buying food for binge-eating episodes as well as the fact that she has had to pay for expensive dental work as a result of the impact of vomiting on her teeth.

Case Example: Jackie

Jackie is now 41, but her eating disorder symptoms started in adolescence when she developed AN as a 14-year-old during the summer after her parents were divorced. She remembers dieting, exercising, weighing herself constantly, and writing down everything she ate. Focusing on her eating was a way to avoid her sadness and anger over her parents' divorce. Jackie did not binge eat or vomit because she would have seen that as "weakness" at a time when she valued self-control over everything else. She recalls feeling terrified of weight gain, even a fraction of a pound, and would weigh herself multiple times a day to make sure her weight was stable. Concerned about her weight loss, her parents had her hospitalized in a local eating disorder program where she was diagnosed with AN. Gradually, Jackie resumed her normal eating patterns, was discharged from the hospital, and saw a therapist for 6 months to ensure that she was continuing to improve, which she did. Although Jackie noticed occasional body image problems (e.g., that her "thighs looked huge"), she was free from eating disorder symptoms throughout high school and college.

After graduation, she started working as a laboratory technician in a company where she was employed for several decades. She had a number of friends at work but generally regarded herself as a shy person and rarely dated. At a professional conference 3 years ago, however, she met her current husband. After they met, she left her job and moved out of state so they could live in the same city. They were married 2 years ago, and Jackie gave birth to their son 1 year ago. Soon after giving birth, Jackie had some mild postpartum depression symptoms and decided to "get back in shape" to "look good and feel better" about herself. She began an intense workout routine and a more restrictive diet. She enjoyed taking care of her son but looked forward to his naps so that she could exercise in their basement, which she did for several hours each day. Jackie found that she became increasingly preoccupied with her weight and shape. Although she could still care for her son, she was often distracted and planning her meals and workouts. After a sleep-deprived night in which her infant son was ill, Jackie finally got him to sleep after her husband left for work one morning. Exhausted, but heading to the basement to exercise anyway, she saw a loaf of bread on the counter, noticed how hungry she was, and started to eat a piece. Unable to stop eating once she had started, she ended up eating the entire loaf and felt so full and afraid of gaining weight that she self-induced vomiting. After this initial episode, her bulimic symptoms increased in frequency, and soon Jackie was binge eating and purging whenever she felt overwhelmed by the demands of parenting. She also weighed herself multiple times a day and spent hours trying on clothes that used to fit before the pregnancy. Concerned about how her bulimic symptoms might affect her young son, Jackie asked her ob-gyn for an eating disorder treatment referral. She expressed frustration, stating, "I thought having an eating disorder was something that I got over as a teenager. I can't believe that I'm over 40 and completely obsessed again with my weight."

As these examples portray, people of all ages and personality types are vulnerable to developing bulimic symptoms. The conditions that lead to the development of BN often differ from factors that maintain the disorder. Although BN is known for its behavioral features, particularly binge eating and purging, it is a condition that is associated with debilitating psychological preoccupation with food, shape, and weight, impairment in relationships as well as work and school performance, physical problems, and mood dysregulation. In addition, although individuals who struggle with BN may eventually seek treatment because of these associated problems, they are often ambivalent about change because of the function of their symptoms for mood regulation and their perception that their compensatory behaviors are essential for weight regulation.

Chapter 2

How Bulimia Nervosa
Is Conceptualized in ICAT-BN

Two models of BN, one for onset, one for maintenance, inform the ICAT-BN approach to treatment. These models attempt to integrate a broad array of emotional, interpersonal, and cognitive factors thought to increase the risk of developing and maintaining behaviors associated with BN. The ICAT-BN models differ from other cognitive and interpersonal models underlying treatments for BN (e.g., Agras, 1991; Fairburn et al., 1993b; Fairburn, 1997, 2008) in that there is a greater emphasis on the integration of interpersonal problems, self-evaluation, self-regulation, emotional experience, and, in the case of the ICAT-BN maintenance model, momentary behavioral processes. Because of the significant emphasis on emotional regulation in the ICAT-BN model, contemporary emotion theories (e.g., Gross, 1998; Campos, Frankel, & Camras, 2004; Gratz & Roemer, 2004) are particularly relevant, especially the multidimensional model of emotion regulation by Gratz and Roemer (2004) and its recent application to the understanding of eating disorder behavior (Lavender et al., 2015).

THE ICAT-BN MODEL OF ONSET

In its simplest form, the ICAT-BN model of onset (see Figure 2.1) posits that life experiences (e.g., interpersonal criticism, social comparison, rejection, loss) together with temperamental predispositions (e.g., harm avoidance, negative urgency) contribute to three broad risk factors for emotional difficulties: interpersonal difficulties, a tendency for negative self-evaluation, and self-regulation deficits. Although individual difference variables (e.g. interpersonal experiences, personality traits) are

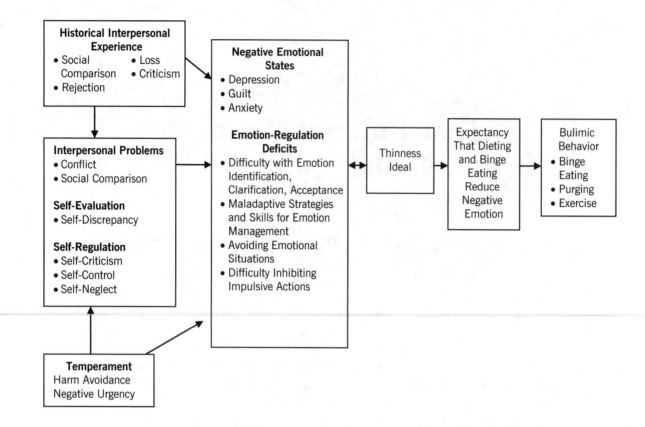

FIGURE 2.1. ICAT-BN model of onset.

considered important background variables in ICAT-BN, they are somewhat de-emphasized in the models because the treatment focuses more explicitly on proximal risks of BN behavior, such as interpersonal difficulties, self-evaluation, and self-regulation deficits. Readers who are interested in a broader model of onset and maintenance of BN that more fully incorporates such individual difference variables and is consistent with ICAT-BN may be interested in reading a recent paper by Pearson, Wonderlich, and Smith (in press).

The ICAT model posits that individuals who experience emotion dysregulation and maintain a strong thinness ideal and expectation that bulimic behavior may reduce distress are thought to be at a particularly heightened risk of BN behavior. Importantly, each of these factors represents a predisposition or characteristic of the BN-prone person. That is, the ICAT-BN onset model suggests that people with elevations on these characteristics may be at increased risk of developing BN. As will be seen in the next section, the maintenance model does not emphasize such individual difference variables, but instead focuses on momentary experiences or processes to explain the function of BN behavior for the person. Next we will review each of the characteristics thought to increase the risk of developing BN in the ICAT-BN model: interpersonal difficulties, negative self-evaluation, self-regulation deficits, negative emotional states, emotion-regulation deficits, thinness ideal, eating-related expectancies, and bulimic behaviors.

Interpersonal Difficulties

The first broad risk factor for emotional disturbance relates to the interpersonal and social stresses (e.g., work, school, or personal relationships) that individuals with BN may experience. Research findings suggest that individuals with BN display significant elevations in a variety of historical interpersonal stresses, including child maltreatment (Welch & Fairburn, 1996; Wonderlich, Brewerton, Jocic, Dansky, & Abbott, 1997) and being raised by parents with psychopathology, including depression and substance abuse (Fairburn, Welch, & Doll, 1997). Previous research also indicates that individuals with BN often perceive their relationships with their parents and their family environments as conflicted, disengaged, and non-nurturing (Kendler et al., 1991; Strober & Humphrey, 1987; Wonderlich, 1992). Observational studies of the families of individuals with BN in the laboratory have supported such findings and suggest that relationships in families of individuals with BN can be described as disengaged, conflicted, and lacking in effective communication (Humphrey, 1986, 1987, 1989). Furthermore, there is evidence that individuals with BN often have personality traits (e.g., low cooperativeness, neuroticism; Cassin & von Ranson, 2005), and we would suggest negative urgency (the tendency to act impulsively when distressed; Pearson et al., in press) that are likely associated with interpersonal difficulties. Of particular significance to the ICAT-BN model is that these interpersonal difficulties are thought to pose a particular risk for affect dysregulation, which in turn increases the risk of bulimic behavior.

Negative Self-Evaluation

The second broad risk for emotional disturbance in the ICAT-BN model is negative self-evaluation (e.g., high self-discrepancy). Previous research suggests that negative self-evaluation serves as a risk factor for bulimic behavior (Fairburn et al., 1997). Individuals with BN also report high levels of perfectionism, particularly maladaptive forms of perfectionism such as doubts about actions and concerns about mistakes (Bardone-Cone et al., 2007). In ICAT-BN, a specific type of negative self-evaluation (i.e., self-discrepancy) is particularly relevant to the onset of BN. Self-discrepancy theory implies that it is not the simple negative perception of the self that is most relevant to BN, but more specifically, the disparity between the perception of one's actual self and one's evaluative standards. These hypotheses are derived from self-discrepancy theory (Higgins, 1987) and its application to depression (Strauman,

1989a,b; Vieth et al., 2003) as well as to eating disorder behaviors (Strauman, Vookles, Berenstein, Chaiken, & Higgins, 1991; Strauman & Glenberg, 1994).

Self-discrepancy theory postulates various domains of the self, including the *actual* self (i.e., a mental representation of the attributes or features the individual believes he or she actually possesses), the *ideal* self (i.e., a representation of the attributes that the individual or significant other would ideally like him or her to possess), and the *ought* self (a representation of the attributes that the individual or a significant other believes it is his or her obligation or duty to possess; Strauman et al., 1991). Central to the ICAT-BN perspective are Strauman's findings (Strauman et al., 1991; Strauman & Glenberg, 1994) suggesting that self-discrepancies are related to negative mood, body dissatisfaction, body size overestimation, and bulimic symptoms. Furthermore, Altabe and Thompson (1996) conducted a series of experiments suggesting that appearance-related actual–ideal discrepancy appears to function as an underlying cognitive schema that can influence information processing and impact negative mood in individuals with eating disorders.

Several recent investigations have tested the self-discrepancy component of the ICAT-BN model (e.g. Wonderlich et al., 2008). In two independent studies, individuals with BN were shown to have significantly higher levels of both actual–ideal and actual–ought discrepancies than control subjects. Furthermore, self-discrepancies were shown to be predictive of higher levels of negative mood in both bulimic and control participants. In addition, the relationship between self-discrepancy and BN was mediated by significant elevations in negative mood states, thus empirically supporting the hypothesis that self-discrepancy is related to negative emotion in BN.

Self-Regulation Deficits

The third broad risk factor for emotional disturbance in the ICAT-BN model of onset pertains to deficits in self-regulation (e.g., increased self-criticism and self-control and deficits in self-acceptance). Individuals with BN are posited to be highly critical of any perceived self-deficits, including appearance or performance (Wonderlich, Klein, & Council, 1996; Wonderlich et al., 2008). While such maladaptive self-regulation strategies are thought to increase negative affect, they may also be seen as a response to negative affect (e.g., disappointment or dejection) regarding the person's perceived performance or appearance. In this regard, self-criticism and self-control efforts may be construed as efforts to correct a perception of a "defective self" (Wonderlich et al., 2008). Similarly, low levels of self-acceptance may function to promote continued efforts to improve performance or appearance. Finally, some individuals with BN are thought to engage in a self-neglectful self-regulation pattern. These behaviors seem to reflect a sense of giving up or not protecting the self. This type of behavior may also be seen in instances in which the individual exposes him- or herself to high-risk situations that have proven problematic for the individual in the past (e.g., extremely restricted eating, negative social situations).

Negative Emotional States

Central to ICAT-BN theory is the idea that the previously described relationship problems, self-evaluation deficits, and maladaptive self-regulation increase negative emotion (see Figure 2.1), which, in turn, increases the chance of bulimic behavior. The idea that individuals with BN experience such negative affect has been empirically supported for years (e.g., Davis, Freeman & Garner, 1988; Johnson & Larson, 1982; Ruderman & Grace, 1987). Also, consistent with escape theory (Heatherton & Baumeister, 1991), individuals with BN are believed to experience prolonged states of aversive, self-oriented cognitive preoccupation focused on their perceived self-deficits. Prolonged states of this type of self-awareness and negative self-evaluation may be associated with the high levels of mood and anxiety problems among individuals with BN (Strober & Katz, 1988; Wonderlich & Mitchell, 1997), particularly the negative emotional states of worrying, rumination, and guilt (Berg et al., 2013; Cooper & Fairburn, 1986).

Thus, individuals with BN may experience heightened negative emotion and, in the face of such negative emotion, have difficulty regulating eating behavior. Supporting this idea, recent EMA studies suggest that high negative emotion and low positive emotion precede bulimic behavior (Engel et al., 2007; Haedt-Matt & Keel, 2011). For example, Smyth et al. (2007) found a significant increase in negative emotions in the 4 to 6 hours preceding bulimic behavior and a complementary decrease in negative emotions in the hours following bulimic behavior, suggesting that the rise in negative emotion served as a trigger and that the bulimic behavior functioned to regulate or reduce negative emotion (see Figure 2.2). These findings support the premise that increased states of negative emotion may serve as a significant antecedent or trigger for bulimic behavior and that bulimic behavior may have self-regulating and negative reinforcing properties, which may explain maintenance of bulimic behavior in the context of negative emotion. However, additional time-sensitive studies are needed to clarify these relationships more completely (Haedt-Matt & Keel, 2011).

Emotion-Regulation Deficits

ICAT-BN theory posits that it is not simply high levels of negative emotional experience that precipitate bulimic behaviors, but that individuals with BN display deficits in their strategies for regulating such emotions and that these deficits play a prominent role in eliciting bulimic behaviors. Although several theories of affect

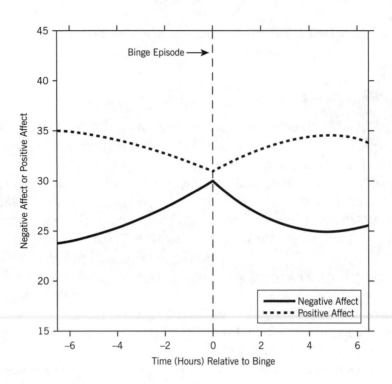

FIGURE 2.2. Negative affect and binge eating. From Smyth et al. (2007). Copyright 2007 by the American Psychological Association. Reprinted by permission.

regulation significantly impacted ICAT-BN's development (Farach & Mennin, 2007; Selby, Anestis, & Joiner, 2008; Cyders & Smith, 2010), the multidimensional model of emotion regulation by Gratz and Roemer (2004) has had a particular impact on ICAT-BN theory. Gratz and Roemer's theory posits that emotion dysregulation can be characterized by deficits in the following areas: (1) identifying and experiencing emotional states, (2) adaptive strategies and skills for managing emotion, (3) the ability to inhibit impulsive behaviors in the face of negative emotional states, and (4) difficulties approaching emotion-eliciting cues. A recent review of the literature examining emotion regulation deficits in individuals with eating disorders suggests that individuals with BN display deficits in all four of Gratz and Roemer's emotion-regulation dimensions (Lavender et al., 2015). Given these emotion-regulation deficits, the ICAT-BN model posits that individuals with BN attempt to engage in a variety of interpersonal and self-directed coping behaviors as attempts to regulate emotion, but these efforts either are ineffective or exacerbate negative emotion. Consequently, individuals with BN may rely on more extreme behavior such as dieting, binge eating, or purging to regulate emotional intensity.

Thinness Ideal

Consistent with previous findings (Striegel-Moore, Silbertstein, & Rodin, 1986), there is evidence that the internalization of the thinness ideal of Western society may be a specific risk factor for eating pathology (Stice, 2002). Internalization of the thinness ideal has been found to correlate with eating problems and body image disturbance (Stice, Schupak-Neuberg, Shaw, & Stein, 1994; Thompson, Heinberg, Altabe, & Tantleff-Dunn, 1999), as well as predict the development of body dissatisfaction (Stice, 2001) and bulimic symptoms among adolescent females (Stice & Agras, 1998). From the ICAT-BN perspective, pursuit of the thinness ideal may be construed as a strategy to attempt to reduce self-discrepancy, but it is a strategy that often leads to an increase in bulimic behavior, given that pursuit of a thin ideal is likely to ultimately increase self-discrepancy and associated negative affect.

Eating-Related Expectancies

Another important element of the ICAT-BN model is that individuals with BN come to expect that eating disorder symptoms will be helpful, particularly in terms of relieving negative emotional states. While both individuals with AN and BN expect that dieting will be beneficial for them, individuals with BN differ from those with AN, as well as those without eating disorders, in expecting that binge eating will help alleviate negative emotional states (Hohlstein, Smith, & Atlas, 1998). Furthermore, individuals who expect that eating may serve beneficial functions in terms of emotion regulation are more likely to experience binge eating during adolescence (Smith, Simmons, Flory, Annus, & Hill, 2007; Pearson, Combs, Zapolski, & Smith, 2012) and during college (Fischer, Peterson, & McCarthy, 2013).

Bulimic Behaviors

In the ICAT-BN model, bulimic behaviors are thought to be elicited by negative emotions as well as expectancies that BN behaviors will reduce negative emotions. However, they are also posited to reciprocally modify such emotions and provide a reward in the form of negative reinforcement. Furthermore, this rewarding emotion-regulation function of bulimic behaviors is believed to be a central factor in the maintenance of BN. The powerful negative reinforcement provided by bulimic symptoms has important clinical implications. By the time an individual with BN seeks treatment, regardless of the cause of BN behaviors, the negatively reinforcing maintenance factors have been established. For this reason, ICAT-BN targets these maintenance factors, rather than etiological mechanisms that may not serve a maintenance function. We will review the ICAT-BN maintenance model next.

THE ICAT-BN MAINTENANCE MODEL

Establishing a maintenance model that is distinct from a model of onset is important both scientifically and clinically (Stice, 2002). Many of the factors that contribute to the etiology of BN may have little to do with the maintenance of the disorder. Consider the example of dieting as a precursor to BN. Dieting is considered a significant risk factor for eating disorders, and most etiological models and clinical formulations of BN include dieting as a factor in the development of this disorder. However, for some individuals with BN, the significance of dieting in the maintenance of the disorder may be less significant than it was for the onset, and other factors (e.g., negative reinforcement in the context of reduced distress) may sustain the behavior. In the ICAT-BN maintenance model (see Figure 2.3) we have attempted to identify a core process that we believe operates to sustain the disorder, regardless of the nature of its origin. Furthermore, we believe the maintenance model is particularly important to clinicians who are interacting with individuals who have already developed BN. While understanding factors that contributed to the onset of BN may be helpful in conceptualizing any case, we believe targeting maintenance factors is most likely to produce beneficial outcomes, which is why the maintenance model is emphasized in ICAT-BN treatment.

This model emphasizes explicit types of triggering situations, emotional responding, and bulimic behaviors. Most important, the model is momentary and relies on brief periods of time in which triggering situations elicit affective states that precipitate bulimic behavior, which in turn modulate the negative affect, thus negatively reinforcing the behavior. Several kinds of triggering situations are thought to be common in BN and parallel the risk factors in the onset model, but in the maintenance model these factors are momentary experiences. The first is best understood as experiences of negative self-evaluation. Specifically, this pertains to situations in

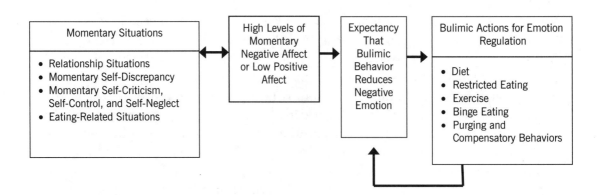

FIGURE 2.3. The ICAT-BN momentary maintenance model.

which the individual with BN appraises him- or herself as not meeting a standard (experiencing self-discrepancy), which leads to increased negative emotion. The second type of situation that may trigger states of negative emotion pertains to explicit behavior reflecting maladaptive self-regulation, such as moments of self-criticism or excessive self-control. Often this process involves harsh, control-oriented behaviors directed toward the self that ultimately result in worsening of negative emotion. The third precipitant of negative emotional states pertains to situations involving interpersonal relationships. ICAT-BN focuses on specific interpersonal problems and situations that clearly precede and precipitate aversive emotional reactions and bulimic behavior. The fourth possible precipitant of emotional reactions is simple exposure to food or efforts to eat in an adaptive and controlled fashion. Some individuals with BN have pronounced emotional dysregulation in response to such food- and eating-related stimuli, which serve as a trigger in the ICAT-BN momentary maintenance model. It is also possible that situational cues, often food related, may trigger BN behavior that is not obviously accompanied by emotional reactions and seems automatic or like a "habit" to the patient (see Chapter 7).

In most bulimic episodes, the individual maintains some type of cognitive expectancy that bulimic behavior (e.g., bingeing, purging) will be helpful in terms of regulating the self, particularly the negative emotional state. As mentioned previously, in the model of onset, bulimic individuals have been demonstrated to maintain the expectancy that bulimic behavior will help them manage negative mood states (Hohlstein et al., 1998). Expecting bulimic behavior to provide some relief from negative emotion is consistent with the functional perspective of ICAT-BN. From this perspective, repeated episodes of bulimic behavior provide learning trials for the individual that result in the expectancy that bulimic behavior may provide some advantage or assistance in terms of the individual's emotional experience. Once this expectancy is established, the presence of negative emotional states may elicit the expectancy, which in turn increases the likelihood of engaging in actual bulimic behavior.

It is crucial to highlight the clinical significance of the momentary nature of the ICAT-BN maintenance model, particularly in terms of clinically examining the time frames surrounding bulimic episodes. The clinical time frame for ICAT-BN will typically not focus on situations and emotions that occurred several weeks or months earlier; rather ICAT-BN is focused on specific episodes of bulimic behavior and the situations and emotions that immediately preceded the episode by moments or hours (ideally). This momentary perspective of the maintenance model has been heavily influenced by EMA research in eating disorders. As described above, these studies strongly suggest that negative emotional states demonstrate a significant and potent influence on the occurrence of bulimic behavior and that bulimic behaviors reduce aversive emotional reactions (e.g., Smyth et al., 2007; Berg et al., 2013). In support of this temporal perspective, recent EMA evidence suggests that following interpersonal and work-related stressful events, individuals with BN experience significant increases in negative affect over a period of hours, which are, in turn, associated with the occurrence of bulimic episodes (Goldschmidt et al., 2013). Overall, EMA data have significantly influenced a framework for understanding BN based on specific episodes of behavior and the triggers and correlates in the brief windows of time preceding them. As a treatment, ICAT-BN attempts to facilitate awareness of the momentary precipitants of bulimic behavior and devise momentary interventions to change actions in response to these precipitants.

THE CASE OF HEIDI

Heidi was a 21-year-old college sophomore when she began treatment for BN. She was raised in a family with two older sisters and her parents. Both of her parents were accomplished professionals, and her father was a long-distance runner while her mother coached the local high school golf team. Both of her sisters were college athletes who also excelled academically and after college obtained prestigious jobs. Heidi was the youngest child in the family by 5 years, and in spite of considerable effort on her part was unable to achieve the level of success of her older sisters. As a result, she perceived her parents as being disappointed in her. She became involved in a summer theater troupe in which she was a valued member of the cast and found this experience both enjoyable and fulfilling. When she was asked to try out for a lead part in a play, she lost 15 pounds in preparation for the role through dieting and exercise. After performing successfully, she attributed her success, in part, to her weight loss. Although she continued to have success in the theater company and obtained increasingly significant acting roles, she also became increasingly anxious about her performances. On a particularly anxiety-ridden evening, she rather impulsively engaged in a binge-eating episode and immediately self-induced vomiting because of fears that she would gain weight. Although Heidi felt a sense of relief after binge–purge episodes, she disliked her bulimic symptoms and felt increasingly preoccupied with eating and appearance. However, she increasingly felt compelled to continue her binge-eating and vomiting behaviors, relying on the "relief" they provided from the mounting pressures she experienced in the context of her theater performances.

In ICAT-BN terminology, Heidi had high standards for herself, particularly based on her sisters' accomplishments, which she believed set a standard she was failing to meet. Importantly, she also believed that she had not met the standards of her parents. This experience produced a significant discrepancy between the perception of her true or actual self and her ideal self. The discrepancy in her self-evaluation elicited moments of strong negative feelings about herself that were initially reduced when she began to participate in the theater. However, as the perceived pressure surrounding her acting performances intensified once she was offered a lead role, her self-discrepancy increased again and she adopted a demanding and controlling self-regulatory style comprised of diet and exercise in an attempt to reduce this self-discrepancy. As the pressures of the theater continued to mount, she experienced increasing levels of stress and anxiety and concerns about performance, which produced emotionally difficult moments that were hard to manage. She learned that binge eating and vomiting provided her with periods of emotional relief. However, binge-eating episodes exacerbated her self-discrepancy because she viewed herself as failing to meet her thinness standards, which had become an important part of her identity, especially in the context of theater.

The case of Heidi highlights how self-discrepancy elicits negative emotional *states*, which in turn, produce *episodes* of binge eating that offer *moments* of relief; ultimately, however, the binge eating results in heightened self-discrepancies and elicits purging behavior. Thus, Heidi offers a prototypical example of the various factors from ICAT-BN theories that may help to explain not only the onset of BN, but also the momentary affect-regulating aspects of bulimic behavior that promote maintenance over time. The structure, goals, and strategies for treating BN with ICAT, which follow from the onset and maintenance models, are discussed next.

Chapter 3

Emotion Focus, Structure, Goals, and Strategies in ICAT-BN

ICAT-BN is a structured, short-term psychological treatment that has been heavily influenced by studies of the relationship of emotion processes and BN behavior. The treatment is oriented around four phases and targets specific goals and objectives. Furthermore, there are several recommended clinical strategies for achieving these goals. While clinicians may make adjustments to the structure or strategies of ICAT-BN for a particular patient, the randomized controlled trial on which the evidence for ICAT-BN is based adhered strictly to these structures, goals, and strategies.

ICAT-BN has been developed for patients who are appropriate candidates for outpatient treatment. Specifically, they should be medically stable and able to engage in an intensive, short-term, structured treatment plan. The presence of psychosis, extreme behavioral instability in multiple domains, or substance use problems may significantly limit the effectiveness of ICAT-BN. Also, ICAT-BN clinicians should have received some degree of specialty training in the delivery of psychotherapy and be both professionally and ethically well suited to the delivery of outpatient mental health treatment. ICAT-BN is optimally delivered by clinicians who have familiarity with short-term structured interventions that encourage direct behavior change, the establishment of behavioral goals, and extensive involvement of the patient in the treatment process, including homework completion. Next, we provide an overview of the emotion-focused base and structure of ICAT-BN, as well as the strategies and techniques that are recommended for pursuing the goals of the treatment.

EMOTION FOCUS OF ICAT-BN

Over the last decade, there has been growing recognition not only that individuals with BN experience intense emotional states such as depression and anxiety, but also that these negative emotional states may figure prominently in the occurrence of individual episodes of bulimic behavior. This observation emerges frequently in EMA studies of individuals with eating disorders. These studies require individuals to carry portable handheld electronic devices (e.g., personal digital assistants, cell phones) that are designed to collect intensive, longitudinal, momentary data about individuals in the natural environment. Participants in such studies are signaled by the handheld device numerous times per day and asked to report about emotional states, events, and behaviors (including eating disorder behaviors). The result is an extremely rich and intensive diary of information about the lives of individuals with eating disorders and about their experiences as they are actually being lived.

EMA studies of individuals with BN have revealed several interesting observations. For example, individuals with BN appear most likely to engage in bulimic behavior in the late afternoon and early evening. Furthermore, weekends appear to be particularly likely times to engage in binge and purge behaviors (Smyth et al., 2009). Data also suggest that individuals with BN experience different kinds of "emotional days" and that bulimic behavior seems to be more strongly associated with some kinds of days than with others. Individuals with BN are also more likely to engage in bulimic behavior on days when they experience more negative emotion later in the day. Interestingly, on days when high levels of negative emotion are experienced early in the day, but not later in the day, bulimic episodes are not significantly increased (Crosby et al., 2009). These studies also indicate that certain types of stressful events (e.g., work, school, interpersonal) are associated with significant increases in negative emotion in the ensuing hours, which, in turn, is associated with increased rates of binge and purge behavior (Goldschmidt et al., 2014). Finally, evidence also suggests that although several types of negative emotion may be involved in precipitating bulimic episodes, the experience of guilt, or perhaps shame, is particularly potent in terms of eliciting bulimic behavior (Berg et al., 2013).

Although there are many variations in the EMA studies conducted to date, one compelling finding emerges repeatedly: in the hours preceding bulimic behavior, individuals with BN report escalating levels of negative emotions and, typically, decreasing levels of positive emotions. This observation was supported in a large meta-analysis examining the relationship between emotion and behavior in EMA studies of individuals with eating disorders (Haedt-Matt & Keel, 2011). While ICAT-BN targets a variety of different behaviors associated with BN (e.g., binge eating, purging, interpersonal behavior), a central theme throughout the treatment is the importance of emotional states in the occurrence of bulimic episodes and, furthermore, the intentional and direct clinical targeting of those emotional states.

Emotion Regulation and ICAT-BN

Given the potent link between emotion and bulimic behavior, ICAT-BN emphasizes emotions in its conceptualization of bulimic behavior and its overall treatment strategy. This means that ICAT-BN is a treatment that emphasizes awareness of emotional experience, of the situations that elicit strong emotional reactions, and of an individual's action tendencies when they are experiencing negative emotional states. This perspective is consistent with several recent emotion-related theories of eating disorder behavior (e.g., Hatch et al., 2010; Haynos & Fruzzetti, 2011; Wildes, Ringham, & Marcus, 2010), as well as several newer eating disorder treatments that include an emphasis on emotional functioning (e.g., Safer, Telch, & Chen, 2009; Wildes & Marcus, 2011). These developments are in line with a growing emphasis on the concept of emotion regulation and its relevance to the broader realm of psychopathology (e.g., Rottenberg & Johnson, 2007; Lewis, Haviland-Jones, & Barrett, 2008). In its simplest form, emotion regulation involves what people do to regulate emotional experiences (e.g., Gross, 1998). Applications to psychopathology typically imply that the behaviors or symptoms of various psychopathological conditions reflect efforts to regulate underlying negative emotional experiences. For example, borderline personality disorder (Gratz, Rosenthal, Tull, Lejuez, & Gunderson, 2006), substance use disorder (Fox, Axelrod, Paliwal, Sleeper, & Sinha, 2007), nonsuicidal self-injury (Muehlenkamp et al., 2009), and, more recently, eating disorders (Haynos & Fruzzetti, 2011) have all been conceptualized as disorders of emotion regulation.

The study of emotion regulation is expanding rapidly, and numerous relevant themes or debates are evolving. For example, a common idea in emotion-regulation theory is that negative emotion in and of itself does not predict psychopathology—rather it is the individual's ability to respond to and regulate underlying emotions (Gratz, 2007). There is also debate in the emotion-regulation literature over whether emotion regulation involves the effort to control emotions or to control behavior when experiencing emotions. Gratz (2007) suggests that in effective emotion regulation, negative emotions are not controlled, but instead accepted as a part of normal emotional experience and that effective regulation involves controlling maladaptive behaviors when experiencing such emotions. Other debates involve the degree to which emotion regulation involves implicit versus explicit processes (Gyurak, Gross, & Etkin, 2011), as well as intrapersonal versus interpersonal processes (Campos, Walle, Dahl, & Main, 2011; Thompson, 1994). There is also uncertainty about whether emotion and emotion regulation are best conceptualized as reflecting a single unified process (i.e., a one-factor model), in which emotion regulation is inherent and occurs throughout the process of emotional experience, or as a discrete process (i.e., a two-factor model) in which emotions are generated by one process and regulated by another (e.g., Gross & Feldman-Barrett, 2011; Kappas, 2011).

While all of these issues are scientifically interesting, their direct applicability to the development of a treatment such as ICAT-BN is somewhat difficult to ascertain. Gratz and Roemer (2004) have developed a clinically relevant multidimensional model of emotion regulation that is directly applicable to a treatment such as ICAT-BN. They posit that effective emotion regulation comprises four fundamental dimensions:

1. Emotional awareness, clarity, and acceptance.
2. Flexible use of adaptive strategies to modulate (vs. eliminate) the intensity and/or temporal features of emotional response.
3. Resisting impulsive behaviors and maintaining the ability to engage in goal-directed behaviors in the context of emotional distress.
4. A willingness to experience emotional distress in the context of pursuing meaningful activities.

This model draws heavily on the theory of Thompson (1994), particularly in terms of emotion regulation serving the function of obtaining goals and also in the theory's emphasis on modulating emotional states rather than attempting to control or eliminate these experiences. To date, the various dimensions of this model have been studied in relation to numerous forms of psychopathology, including substance use disorders (e.g., Fox et al., 2007; Fox, Hong, & Sinha, 2008), borderline personality disorder (e.g., Bornovalova et al., 2008; Gratz et al., 2006), anxiety disorders (e.g., Mennin, McLaughlin, & Flanagan, 2009; Roemer et al., 2009), nonsuicidal self-injury (e.g., Gratz & Tull, 2010; Muehlenkamp et al., 2009), and impulse control disorders, including compulsive buying and pathological gambling (e.g., Williams, Grisham, Erskine, & Cassedy, 2012; Williams & Grisham, 2012). Within this framework, deficits in one or more of the dimensions are conceptualized as being indicative of emotion dysregulation and are thus theorized to function as potential etiological or maintaining factors for psychopathology.

Recently, Lavender et al. (2015) have reviewed the relevant emotion-focused literature on BN in terms of the four dimensions of Gratz and Roemer's model. Application of these dimensions to BN revealed that individuals with BN experience deficits in all four of Gratz and Roemer's dimensions of emotion regulation. That is, individuals with BN display a decreased awareness and acceptance of emotions; deficits in adaptive emotion-regulation strategies; and difficulties in the inhibition of impulsive behaviors during times of emotional distress. In addition, individuals with BN may avoid important activities due to the anticipation of negative emotional states associated with such activities (including eating). The results of this review support the fundamental idea that BN is associated with significant emotion-regulation deficits and that the use of emotion-focused interventions to treat this condition is scientifically supported.

Working with Emotion in ICAT-BN

The idea that individuals with BN experience significant emotion-regulation problems is associated with several practical features of ICAT-BN. First, there is a clear emphasis in ICAT-BN on the idea that negative emotional experiences are a natural and understandable aspect of life that cannot be suppressed or avoided effectively; rather, ICAT-BN emphasizes attempting to help patients control behavior during significant negative emotional states. Second, there is a pervasive emphasis throughout ICAT-BN on improving awareness of emotional responses, their origins, and urges for action in the face of various emotional states. Third, ICAT-BN emphasizes acquiring skills to help control or restrain behaviors in the face of negative emotion. This may include tolerating emotional states, careful plans for adaptive responding, and efforts to inhibit impulsive or rash actions in response to emotional cues. Fourth, ICAT-BN emphasizes attempting to identify sources of emotion dysregulation and encourage direct efforts to modify these cues or exposure to them. Each of these strategies will be discussed throughout Chapters 5–8 as we highlight the implementation of ICAT-BN through the four phases of treatment.

ICAT-BN TREATMENT STRUCTURE

ICAT-BN is designed to be conducted over a minimum of 21 sessions, each approximately 45–50 minutes in length. In the primary randomized controlled trial of ICAT-BN (Wonderlich et al., 2014), the treatment was precisely 21 sessions, in large part to make it directly comparable to CBT-E for research purposes. The complexities of clinical practice may necessitate shorter or longer versions of ICAT-BN. Clinicians can adjust the duration of treatment while balancing the need to maintain fidelity to the original treatment model and meet the needs of an individual patient.

ICAT-BN is delivered across four different phases. Each phase has a broad, general purpose; several topics may be addressed within each phase (see Table 3.1). Phase I emphasizes enhancing motivation, engaging in the treatment, and education about BN from an ICAT perspective. In a 21-session treatment, Phase I typically lasts two to four sessions. It is recommended that sessions be conducted twice a week until Phase II is completed. This results in Phase I being completed within 1 or 2 weeks. Phase II begins with a direct emphasis on modifying eating behavior and habits surrounding meals and snacks. In Phase II, the clinician works with the patient to begin to make concrete changes in the planning, purchasing, preparation, and consumption of meals without purging. Typically, Phase II will last six to eight sessions or up to the eighth or ninth session of treatment.

Phase III of ICAT-BN focuses on identifying and modifying precipitants of negative emotional states. There are four broad areas of emotion dysregulation that

TABLE 3.1. Summary of ICAT Phases

Phase of ICAT	Treatment strategies	Specific interventions
Phase I: Introduction and Motivation	1. Motivational enhancement. 2. Psychoeducation. 3. Emotion education.	1. Examine impact of current bulimic behavior on broader goals for life. 2. Self-monitor food intake and context. 3. FEEL skill.
Phase II: Nutritional Rehabilitation	1. Meal planning and food logs. 2. Identify emotions associated with eating. 3. Develop adaptive coping strategies for urge control. 4. Identify factors associated with avoidance or lack of uptake of CARE skill.	1. Encourage meal plan and regular consumption of meals/ snacks (CARE skill) conjointly with goal setting (GOAL skill). 2. Continue use of FEEL skill. 3. Actively teach coping skills for purpose of managing urges through the ACT skill. 4. Review CARE plan results. 5. Elicit and monitor affect throughout CARE planning.
Phase III: Interpersonal Patterns, Self-Directed Styles, and Self-Discrepancy	1. Initial formulation and collaborative decision about behavioral target for Phase III. 2. Determine if relationship problems are present and recurrent. 3. Consider how self-regulation behavior may be related to bulimic behavior. 4. Address role that self-evaluation (i.e., self-discrepancy) may play in bulimic behavior. 5. Use GOAL skill to focus change in relevant area. 6. Continue meal planning and food monitoring.	1. Continue use of FEEL, GOAL, CARE, and ACT skills. 2. Utilize SEA Change Diaries to identify types of situations that trigger bulimic episodes (e.g., relationships, self-regulation, self-evaluation, and food related). 3. Use skills to address relationship problems (SAID), self-regulation problems (SPA), or self-evaluation issues (REAL).
Phase IV: Relapse Prevention	1. Develop Healthy Lifestyle Plan. 2. Develop written relapse prevention plan. 3. Promote vigilance and coping perspective for slip management. 4. Address feelings related to termination.	1. Review progress in treatment. 2. Formalize relapse prevention plan and healthy lifestyle strategies. 3. Introduce WAIT skill. 4. Elicit and monitor affect.

are commonly addressed in Phase III: (1) interpersonal problems, (2) self-evaluation problems, (3) self-regulation problems, and (4) food- and eating-related triggers of negative emotions. The clinician and patient formulate the focus of Phase III through collaborative goal-setting sessions at the beginning of the phase. Phase III typically lasts 11–12 sessions, depending on the length of Phase II. Finally, Phase IV emphasizes relapse prevention and general lifestyle modifications. It typically consists of the final two to three sessions of ICAT-BN.

Throughout all four phases of ICAT-BN, there is an emphasis on eight core skills. Each of these skills is designed to represent a core behavioral process considered a key aspect of recovery and is actively included in ICAT treatment sessions. The skills are referred to by the following acronyms (skill domain in parentheses): FEEL (emotion awareness), CARE (meal planning), GOAL (goal setting), ACT (coping with urges), SAID (interpersonal skills), SPA (adaptive self-regulation), REAL (realistic self-evaluation), and WAIT (impulse control). These skills are described in more detail in Chapter 4, including Table 4.1.

Each phase of ICAT-BN treatment is accompanied by a collection of handouts, which patients are encouraged to take home and complete outside of sessions as a component of their treatment (see Figure 3.1). Patients are asked to practice core skills, complete self-monitoring forms, and perform other therapeutic tasks in order to generalize skills and provide momentary data for treatment sessions. Recommended handouts and copies of the eight skill cards are included in Part III of this book.

Clearly, clinicians will need to use their own judgment in applying certain aspects of the treatment depending on the needs of specific patients. For example, some patients may require modifications in the length of particular phases. Additionally, some patients may experience situations that trigger negative emotions that are not fully articulated in ICAT but deserve attention. Furthermore, there will be variation in the degree to which the ICAT-BN model appears to fit a given individual's experience. Part II of this book, which describes how to carry out Phases I–IV of ICAT-BN, is not meant to be a prescriptive protocol that must be followed precisely in all cases; instead, it aims to provide a broad perspective on the use of ICAT-BN to treat bulimic symptoms, with an emphasis on clinical utility.

TREATMENT GOALS

Two fundamental objectives of ICAT are to (1) reduce use of bulimic behaviors in high-risk moments and (2) enhance emotion-regulation skills to manage situations that trigger emotion dysregulation and drive bulimic behaviors. This first objective is clearly addressed in Phase II as the patient begins to restore more normative eating and begins to manage urges to engage in bulimic behavior. The second objective is

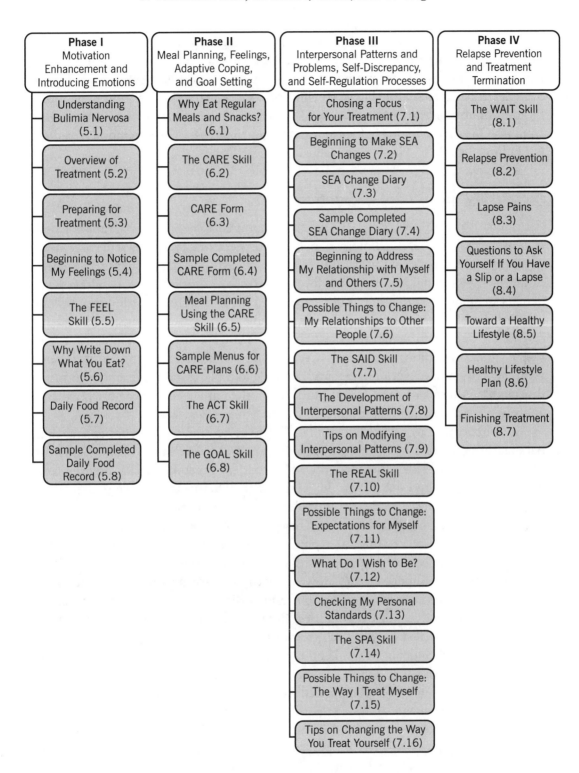

FIGURE 3.1. Participant handouts by treatment phase.

largely addressed in Phase III as the patient attempts to identify and modify factors that precipitate negative emotional states. Thus, it may be useful for clinicians to recognize that Phase II places a particular emphasis on increased behavioral control over eating behaviors while Phase III emphasizes more effective emotion regulation. In addition to these broad goals, several other more specific objectives are emphasized in ICAT-BN, which if achieved are thought to increase the likelihood of reducing bulimic behavior. These are reviewed next.

Increasing Awareness of Emotion

An essential principle of ICAT-BN is that emotional experience is a fundamental part of the biology and psychology of people. Furthermore, emotions will sometimes be positive and often be negative. ICAT-BN theory assumes that a lack of awareness of negative emotional states or low levels of positive emotional states, along with deficits in emotion-regulation skills, can increase the likelihood of bulimic behavior. Rather than attempting to suppress or deny emotional reactions, ICAT-BN is oriented toward increasing awareness of such feelings and facilitating a full experience of such reactions. However, ICAT-BN does not simply focus on increasing awareness of aversive emotional states, but aims to understand these emotions more thoroughly in terms of their origins and assists the patient in finding effective and adaptive ways to manage these states.

It is important to acknowledge that the range of emotional experiencing that patients bring to treatment or can acquire from treatment varies dramatically. In our studies, we have identified patients who experience their emotions intensely and genuinely, both in and out of session. Many of these patients are able to articulate their emotional experience clearly and tolerate the examination of these states, their origins, and the associated action tendencies. In such cases, the ICAT-BN clinician will work to deepen the emotional experience and heighten awareness with the idea that this will enhance the skill capabilities of the patient to regulate emotional states in the future without binge eating. However, we have also encountered patients who seem to be able to acknowledge emotions and perhaps even label them, but deeper exploration of these feelings was limited either by the patient's introspective skills or by a seeming wish to avoid such examination. In some cases, careful emotion facilitation by the clinician expanded the patient's emotional awareness and level of experiencing, but this was not always true. Some patients seemed content to simply acknowledge that emotions were indeed important, and they attempted to identify them in the environment and manage them without significantly experiencing the emotional state. Other patients did not attempt to identify or experience emotions, but this response appeared to be part of a broader pattern of disengagement or extreme ambivalence about treatment. Thus, in spite of the fact that ICAT-BN is an emotionally focused treatment, it needs to be acknowledged that the awareness, experiencing, and identification of emotions will likely vary both in quality and quantity among patients, and such variability should be carefully considered in the delivery of ICAT-BN.

Modifying Emotion–Action Units

One of the fundamental tenets of ICAT-BN is that individuals with BN have significant problems regulating emotional states and that their eating disorder symptomatology serves as an emotion-regulation strategy. Modifying emotional states and their influence on BN behavior is a clear objective of ICAT-BN. During Phases I and II, the clinician and patient begin to develop skills in the area of emotion recognition as well as an understanding of the relationship between emotions and BN behavior. Early in Phase I, patients begin to monitor, identify, and label emotional states both within and outside of the session. Such emotional states are carefully examined to determine how they may precipitate bulimic behaviors, and how binge eating and purging (as well as other compensatory behaviors) may serve to regulate them. Later in treatment, as the clinician and patient begin to identify the role of emotions that precipitate bulimic behaviors, there is also a search for the function of the bulimic behavior. For example, does the patient expect that the behavior will provide a way to avoid or escape negative states? Do bulimic behaviors allow a temporary distraction from a distressing situation? Do the behaviors enhance positive emotion? Increasing awareness of these possibilities results in an emphasis on finding alternative, adaptive behaviors that may serve the same function as the bulimic behaviors and meet underlying needs (e.g., need for distraction or distress reduction) in a more adaptive fashion. To this end, skills are introduced to promote goal setting, adaptive coping, and reduction in bulimic behavior.

Identifying Situations That Trigger Emotion–Action Units

A fundamental objective in ICAT-BN is the identification of triggers of negative emotions. Thus clinicians attempt to identify and modify the source of the emotion dysregulation that is associated with the bulimic behavior. The clinician and patient work together to identify the situations, events, and personal experiences that precede negative emotions and subsequent bulimic behaviors. Most often, these emotions emerge from the four broad categories of triggers outlined in the ICAT-BN maintenance model: (1) interpersonal relationships and external stressors (e.g., school, work); (2) negative self-evaluation (e.g., not meeting personal standards); (3) maladaptive self-regulatory behaviors (e.g., self-criticism); and (4) emotionally related urges cued by the presence of food or eating. ICAT-BN directly intervenes to attempt to modify these high-risk precipitants and reduce the overall level of negative affect that is believed to trigger bulimic behavior.

STRATEGIES FOR ACHIEVING THE GOALS AND OBJECTIVES OF ICAT-BN

The goals and objectives of ICAT-BN are pursued through a variety of strategies or approaches to treatment. These strategies include utilization of core skills, direct modification of eating behavior, functional analysis that examines situations, emotions, and actions, and emphasis on maintaining a momentary focus.

Skills-Based Orientation to Treatment

One of the strategies embedded in ICAT-BN to promote behavioral change is an explicit delineation of the eight core skills thought to underlie recovery from BN, which are outlined more thoroughly in Chapter 4. The eight core skills represent behaviors in various domains, including emotion regulation, eating behavior, interpersonal relationships, urge management, and other behaviors thought to be important for recovery from BN. Each patient will receive an individual formulation of his or her problem, and skills will be incorporated into the formulation to help modify deficits or excesses. Interventions will often include explicit review of the core skills and recommendations for implementing the skills outside of sessions. The focus on the eight core skills is designed to facilitate a consistent theme in an individual's treatment, which is oriented around particular skills deficits that are considered important to the maintenance of his or her BN. However, as discussed in Chapter 4, ICAT-BN is not a simple prescription of skill-based practice. The highly collaborative nature of the treatment and the emphasis on emotional factors in bulimic episodes, and on the various situations in a person's life that trigger emotional difficulties make ICAT-BN a highly personalized and subjectively meaningful treatment. The skills provide an opportunity for the clinician and the patient to maintain a focus on particularly relevant behavioral deficits or excesses and on interventions designed to alleviate them.

Encouraging Modification of Eating Behavior through the CARE Skill

One of the essential skills for all patients is the CARE skill, which is an acronym for Calmly Arrange Regular Eating (see Chapter 4). ICAT-BN includes an explicit focus in Phase II on modifying eating behavior directly through efforts to change the timing, quantity, and quality of eating episodes. This strategy directly and explicitly encourages planful selection, consumption, and retention of food and is considered essential to modify the disordered eating behavior that individuals with BN experience regularly. While some patients find this direct focus on eating distressing, clinicians will try to find ways to encourage the adaptive consumption of food while simultaneously addressing the emotional reaction that patients may have to such an objective change. Importantly, ICAT-BN does not simply provide direction or instruction to "eat more" or "eat differently," but encourages a thorough understanding of the emotional consequences of such change while simultaneously working with the patient to use skills to modify eating episodes, manage emotions, and prevent binge eating and purging.

SEA Change Analyses to Promote Change of Functional Bulimic Behavior

ICAT-BN relies on a technique called "SEA Change," an acronym for situation—emotion—action (SEA) units, which are thought to underlie bulimic behavior. Patients and their clinicians track and log *actions* involving bulimic symptoms (e.g., binge eating, purging, meal skipping, excessive exercise). The treatment then focuses on identifying the *situations* that preceded (and possibly elicited) the episodes and the *emotions* that were associated with the bulimic behavior. The idea behind SEA Change is that individuals with BN are often unaware of the environmental and intrapersonal situations (S) that trigger strong emotions (E) and elicit bulimic action (A). Furthermore, individuals with BN may also lack awareness of the actual emotions involved in the process. It is in the context of SEA Change that clinicians attempt to clarify the function that the bulimic actions serve, such as affect regulation. Alternative ways of meeting these functional needs can then be identified.

To illustrate this concept, consider the case of Brandon, who has significant self-doubts, tends to perceive himself negatively, both in terms of appearance and accomplishments, and intermittently binge-eats and excessively exercises. According to ICAT-BN terminology, Brandon may have significant self-discrepancy problems, meaning that his desired self is significantly different from how he perceives himself. Imagine further that Brandon is dedicated to reaching a goal of being "first chair" in his university band saxophone section. After months of practice, he learns that he will not be first chair, and within a few days he begins excessively exercising and binge eating. In this example, the ICAT-BN clinician can focus on the situation (S: not getting first chair) and the action (A: exercising and binge eating), as well as identifying the intervening emotional reaction (E: dejection, sadness, anger). Working with Brandon to identify, understand, and tolerate such emotional states, as well as identifying the likely underlying self-discrepancy, is a critical step in working with individuals with these types of bulimic precipitants. An additional intervention involves collaborating with Brandon to identify the function of the bulimic behaviors. Was it to avoid the feelings of rejection and disappointment? Was it to block out concerns about self-worth? Was it self-punishment for "failing?" Was it an attempt to "redeem" himself by achieving something else? Ultimately, the patient and clinician collaboratively explore the meaning of the situation, the experience of the emotion, and the function of the action, with the goal of modifying the self-discrepancy, identifying and tolerating the negative emotions, and/or finding a more adaptive way to regulate the patient's distress (for Brandon, the dejection, sadness and anger).

Maintaining a Momentary Focus

Numerous EMA studies of BN (e.g., Smyth et al., 2007; Berg et al., 2013; Goldschmidt et al., 2014) consistently reveal that increases in negative affect and parallel decreases in positive affect occur in the moments and hours preceding binge eating and purging behaviors among individuals with BN. This finding has provided an empirical foundation for the *momentary framework* of ICAT-BN. From moment to moment the treatment focuses on significant actions (i.e., bulimic behavior), precipitating emotional states, and the situations that generate them, as well as the potential function of the symptoms.

For example, in the preceding section, we described Brandon, who after a significant disappointment (i.e., not reaching goal as a saxophonist) engages in bulimic behavior, and we speculated that this behavior could be due to the activation of an underlying self-discrepancy, which prompted strong negative emotions. In turn, we implied that the bulimic behavior regulated the negative emotions. We indicated that "within a few days" of not getting the lead saxophone position in the university band he began to exhibit bulimic behavior. However, if Brandon entered ICAT-BN treatment, the clinician would develop a more momentary focus. Rather than focusing on the weeks or days before the bulimic behaviors, the ICAT-BN clinician is interested in trying to modify specific episodes of bulimic behavior. The operative unit of intervention and change is a single BN action or episode. One episode after another is examined in treatment to clarify the SEA pattern characterizing the patient's eating disorder. Through the SEA Change procedure, the ICAT-BN clinician identifies explicit bulimic actions and focuses the intervention on the momentary situational and emotional correlates of the episode.

To maintain a momentary focus with Brandon, his clinician would explicitly direct attention to a single episode of excessive exercise or binge eating. The episode would be situated in time and place in order to understand the momentary precipitants. The clinician would help the patient to remember each experience in vivid detail, including the situation and emotions that preceded it. A variety of questions and interventions could be used to guide the session—for example:

"Tell me more about when you started thinking about the binge. Were you having urges? How were you imagining the binge?"

The clinician might then ask the patient to describe an earlier period of time before the binge eating—for example:

"Tell me about that morning. What was it like for you? Who else was there? What was going through your mind? Did anything explicit happen that morning that seemed important to you?"

When the situation is clarified, the clinician may then shift to the emotional experience—for example, the clinician can ask:

"So I think I have a better understanding of what was happening that morning, but tell me what you were feeling that morning. Were there specific feelings? What was that like for you? As you began to feel that, what did you notice was going through your mind?"

Finally, the clinician can start to focus on the function of, and the expectations of, the behavior. For example, in the case of Brandon the clinician may comment:

"So, I am beginning to understand what happened and how it impacted you. It sounds like on Saturday you spent a lot of time thinking about not getting the first chair in the band. That experience seemed to bring all sorts of questions into your mind about your self-worth, and it left you feeling unhappy and frustrated and also kind of confused. I understand that, but then tell me how you got to the point of the binge-eating episode. What were you thinking about in terms of how that might help you? What was appealing about it? Did you think in some way it could be helpful?"

These examples highlight the importance of focusing on specific details surrounding the behavior in order to identify situations and emotions, rather than more general patterns (e.g., "Do you tend to binge-eat when you are upset?"). Also, by articulating clearly the patient's expectancies regarding possible functions of the behavior, the clinician and patient may identify alternative strategies to replace the bulimic behavior. This momentary focus is a critical aspect of ICAT-BN and provides the foundation for the content and goals of treatment.

This event-focused, momentary approach to intervention rests on the accumulation and integration of a detailed and repeated analysis of actual bulimic episodes over time, which help to maintain an explicit focus on the problem behavior being targeted in ICAT-BN treatment (i.e., bulimic symptoms), as well as the situational and emotional correlates of these symptoms. From the ICAT-BN perspective, the occurrence of a bulimic episode should be considered *a top priority and focus* of treatment. This awareness helps maintain the relevance of the treatment and its focus on bulimic behavior.

Including Significant Others in Treatment

In the randomized controlled trial of ICAT-BN, significant others were not included in the treatment due to issues related to the research design. However, in clinical practice including significant others is frequently an important clinical strategy. In ICAT-BN, it may be reasonable to include significant others for psychoeducational purposes, such as teaching family members about the ICAT-BN model of treatment. One specific strategy would be to involve significant others when the patient's BN behavior is clearly associated with interpersonal problems that involve the significant other (see Chapter 7). ICAT-BN places a significant emphasis on trying to modify variables that precipitate affect dysregulation, and if a particular relationship seems to trigger this kind of affective experience, it would be clinically appropriate to include significant others as an intervention to try and reduce emotional dysregulation and bulimic behavior.

SUMMARY

ICAT-BN is a treatment that attempts to identify and modify both situational and emotional cues of BN behavior. This treatment may involve direct efforts to modify situations that precede BN behavior and improve regulation skills for emotional antecedents of bulimic behavior. Importantly, ICAT-BN attempts to explicitly identify and address situations that lead to momentary episodes of BN behavior.

Chapter 4

Core Skills and the Therapeutic Alliance in ICAT-BN

Disruption of entrenched bulimic behaviors requires focused and repetitive practice that produces new skills and habits and a lifestyle that protects the patient against continued bulimic behavior. Such a lifestyle is not likely attainable without specific and concrete behavioral changes both in eating behavior and other maintenance factors associated with BN. In ICAT-BN, eight skills have been developed to assist in recovery, each of which represents a potential domain of change in treatment. These skills are discussed in the first part of this chapter. However, ICAT-BN is not simply a collection of skills for patients to practice. It is assumed in ICAT-BN that meaningful symptomatic and behavioral changes are limited in the absence of a truly collaborative treatment relationship and a strong therapeutic alliance. The nature of the therapeutic relationship in ICAT is discussed in detail in the second part of this chapter.

SPECIFIC ICAT-BN SKILLS

The eight core skills taught to patients in ICAT-BN are displayed in Table 4.1, each with its target domain, the phase in which it is typically introduced, its acronym, and the elements in the acronym. Clinicians may introduce skills out of phase in order to introduce the patient to particular topics that are immediately relevant or to review topics later in treatment that have been addressed previously. As Table 4.1 suggests, the skills reflect a broad range of behavioral topics including emotional awareness, meal planning, urge management, adaptive coping, goal setting, interpersonal relationships, self-evaluation, self-regulation, and impulse control.

TABLE 4.1. Core Skills in ICAT-BN

Skill-target domain	Phase	Acronym	Elements in acronym
Emotion Awareness	I	FEEL	Focus, Experience, Examine, and Label
Meal Planning	II	CARE	Calmly Arrange Regular Eating
Coping Behavior for Urges	II	ACT	Adaptive Coping Techniques
Setting Goals to Focus Behavior Change Efforts	II	GOAL	Goals and Objectives Affect Life-Moments
Interpersonal Skills	III	SAID	Sensitively Assert Ideas and Desires
Self-Regulation	III	SPA	Self-Protect and Accept
Expectations for Myself	III	REAL	Realistic Expectations Affect Living
Impulse Control and Relapse Prevention	IV	WAIT	Watch All Impulses Today

Emotional Awareness (FEEL)

Because of the emphasis in ICAT-BN on emotion regulation, this skill set is covered in various patient handouts, and clinicians will typically provide simple instructions on the meaning of emotion and its regulation. Furthermore, in ICAT-BN the exploration of emotion in treatment sessions is clearly relevant to emotional awareness. The FEEL skill (Focus, Experience, Examine, Label) is designed to assist patients in learning to identify and tolerate emotional states as well as to begin to examine the cues and origins of their feelings.

Meal Planning (CARE)

Because individuals with BN often have compromised skills in the area of eating nutritionally healthy meals and snacks, there is an explicit emphasis on acquiring, planning, preparing, and eating food without purging. The CARE skill (Calmly Arrange Regular Eating) emphasizes the importance of anticipating, preparing for, and completing eating episodes in an adaptive fashion rather than allowing urges to influence decisions that may result in binge eating.

Urge Management and Adaptive Coping (ACT)

In addition to promoting emotional awareness and planful eating, ICAT-BN also emphasizes inhibiting maladaptive behaviors and developing more adaptive coping skills. The ACT (Adaptive Coping Technique) skill refers to behavioral management of high-risk bulimic moments, such as emotionally dysregulated situations and intense urge moments. This skill set may involve distraction, problem solving, or self-calming behaviors to prevent urges or habits from being enacted. The ACT skill is often implemented by identifying a short, personalized, idiosyncratic sequence of steps for each patient to use in high-risk, intense-urge moments. It may be useful to think of these skills as tools in a toolbox or a new routine that can be implemented in the face of cues and urges. For example, one patient devised the following ACT plan to use when experiencing urges to binge-eat and purge:

1. If possible, get out of the immediate situation (i.e., leave the room).
2. Use the FEEL skill to assess feeling state and triggers.
3. Take a walk or a bike ride to give myself time to evaluate the triggers and think of an alternative to binge eating and purging.

Setting Goals (GOAL)

It is important in ICAT-BN for patients and clinicians to collaboratively set short-term treatment goals that focus on changes in behavior. Establishing goals focuses the intervention and also helps patients concretely identify the problems they wish to address and the strategies and skills they will need to accomplish their goals. Goal setting serves the additional benefit of facilitating an awareness in both the patient and clinician when goals are met. The GOAL skill (Goals and Objectives Affect Life-Moments) is designed to motivate individuals to remain aware of their immediate goals and strategies during stressful moments. For example, the simple goal of attempting to eat breakfast each day for a week may help patients to not lose sight of such behavioral changes when the complexities and stresses of the world interfere. Typically, goal setting focuses on setting short-term objectives for behavior change. We do not recommend setting goals involving a targeted reduction in BN symptoms (e.g., binge, purge) due to the risk of loss of motivation if such goals are not met. Rather, goals can be set to apply certain skills from session to session with a short-term focus on actions that can be taken to manage urges and prevent bulimic symptoms from occurring.

Interpersonal Skills (SAID)

Given the significant difficulty that many individuals with BN have with relationships, ICAT-BN emphasizes interpersonal skill deficits as possible precipitating factors for bulimic episodes. This domain refers to any problem situation in relationships, including difficulties with assertion, struggles with intimacy, avoidant withdrawal from others, submissive behavior, aggressive hostility, and unrealistic expectations of others. However, the ICAT-BN clinician should focus on interpersonal problems only if they are construed as precipitants of negative emotion associated with BN symptoms. The SAID skill (Sensitively Assert Ideas and Desires) reflects a composite of strategies to facilitate social problem solving, assertion, and self-expression in the interpersonal domain.

Self-Regulation (SPA)

Many patients receiving ICAT-BN benefit from developing new skills in terms of how they relate to themselves. The SPA (Self-Protect and Accept) skill pertains to behaviors patients directs toward themselves, often in an effort to change or regulate the self. Some individuals are exceedingly self-critical, others are highly self-controlling, and others seem to neglect themselves. Such self-directed behaviors (e.g., self-criticism) are often present when a bulimic patient fails to meet a standard (see Self-Evaluation and Expectations for Myself below). Given that many individuals with BN engage in self-directed criticism or excessive self-control when they are disappointed in themselves, the SPA skill focuses on increasing self-acceptance and self-protection.

Self-Evaluation and Expectations for Myself (REAL)

Many individuals with bulimic symptoms hold high personal standards that are extraordinarily difficult to attain. Skills in this area examine patients' expectations for themselves and the value they place on those expectations. These skills also address the core construct of self-discrepancy, which involves differences between how the patient perceives him- or herself compared to how he or she would ideally like to be. The REAL skill (Realistic Expectations Affect Living) is designed to assist patients in identifying unrealistic expectations and developing more adaptive, present-focused expectations that include an awareness of their actual strengths and limitations.

Impulse Control (WAIT)

Consistent with the ACT skill, there is also an explicit emphasis in ICAT-BN on attempting to promote adaptive inhibition of rash and potentially self-harming behaviors, including bulimic behaviors *and* other self-damaging behaviors. The WAIT skill (Watch All Impulses Today) involves helping the patient to be aware of high-risk situations, maladaptive emotional reactions, and urges for impulsive and reckless behavior. These impulsive behaviors are not limited to restrictive eating, binge eating, and purging, but also include other self-damaging behaviors that co-occur in individuals with BN (e.g., substance use, sexual promiscuity, self-harm behaviors). The WAIT skill is often introduced in the final phase of therapy in order to emphasize the importance of continuing to monitor impulses after treatment is over in order to prevent relapse. However, for some individuals with high levels of impulsivity, the WAIT skill may be introduced earlier in treatment to assist in the management of particularly problematic behavioral sequences.

USING THE ICAT-BN SKILLS WITH PATIENTS

The ICAT-BN skills serve several functions. First, they help both the patient and clinician stay focused on eight domains of behavior that are considered important for recovery. In ICAT-BN, treatment should be broadly focused on at least one of these domains at any given point in time. A second practical use of the skills is that they serve as a communication strategy. Patients and clinicians may start to think about problems encountered in terms of the domains of the skills. The following example illustrates how skills can be incorporated into discussions about bulimic behavior cues.

Example Dialogue

CLINICIAN: So tell me more about this binge–purge episode on Saturday afternoon.

PATIENT: I think it had something to do with that REAL skill stuff that you were talking about last time. I got really competitive with my friend, and I felt like I had to be better than her at waterskiing. We were on the boat taking turns waterskiing, and there were these two guys in the boat with us. It seemed like the guys were more interested in her than me, and for some reason I just kind of went nuts with skiing. I started even showing off things I could do on skis that my friend can't do. It was like I was trying to prove something.

CLINICIAN: Yeah, was it like you had to be the best skier? What do you think was driving that?

PATIENT: I don't know. (*pause*) Maybe the guys being there, but also just being good at something.

CLINICIAN: You know, let's talk some more about that. I get the part about maybe thinking that you weren't as good as you felt you needed to be, like somehow not living up to your expectations of yourself. But what about your friend? How did she figure into this?

PATIENT: I think I just wanted to be better, better than her at something. I want to be the best at something. Like if I could show everyone that I was a better skier that would mean something to me and them.

CLINICIAN: Yeah, I think you have identified something important here. I hear the REAL skill piece that you mentioned earlier, and I agree that your expectations of yourself were really important to understand in this situation. But there is another thing we talk a lot about in this treatment, and it's another skill that might be relevant. We call it SPA, which stands for Self-Protect and Accept. It's about how you treat yourself, especially when you are dissatisfied or feeling like you aren't meeting your standards. Let's talk more about what happened on the boat and think together about what you might have been doing to yourself that afternoon.

Identifying explicit skills and helping patients learn the key elements in each can lead patients to practice and rehearse these skills. It is common to ask patients to explicitly practice skills within each session and as homework, as well as to review the handouts to help with skill acquisition. Simply put, the skills in ICAT-BN are designed to focus the treatment, enhance communication, and promote behavioral change.

ICAT-BN SKILLS AS PORTABLE STRATEGIES FOR MANAGING MOMENTS IN TIME

Although the ICAT-BN skills are discussed in sessions and reviewed in detailed patient handouts, the skills are also provided in small skill cards (see Part III). (In our study trial, we laminated the cards for patients to facilitate their use.) Based on feedback we have received in our pilot testing and clinical trials, patients often find these portable cards helpful resources, particularly in generalizing skills outside of therapy sessions. Optimally, clinicians and patients work together collaboratively to find ways for patients to generalize skill acquisition by utilizing these skills in the natural environment. In that regard, the ICAT-BN skill cards may be considered treatment extenders that continue to focus patients on working on particular areas of difficulty or deficit. Clinicians should emphasize the use of the cards to patients and discuss it regularly to help them work on their treatment outside of sessions. Ideally, patients will keep the skill cards at their immediate disposal and refer to them for a review of concrete strategies to be used in the moment when they encounter urges for eating disorder behaviors or situations that may increase emotional distress. Additionally, certain skills, such as FEEL, CARE, or ACT, may be practiced and reviewed on a regular basis. Together, clinicians and patients can examine the patient's experiences using the cards, difficulties utilizing skills in the moment, and successful implementation of the skills. Our aim is to ultimately incorporate technology-based interventions in future versions of ICAT-BN so that patients will be able to access their skill cards through their smartphones. In the meantime, some patients have found that taking photos of the skill cards with their smartphones has provided a portable and highly accessible form of the cards for daily use.

WHAT THE ICAT-BN SKILLS ARE NOT

Finally, it is extremely important for clinicians to understand that ICAT-BN is not simply a collection of skills that patients are asked to rehearse and implement. Such a mechanistic and didactic approach is not consistent with the fundamental tenets of ICAT-BN. Rather, ICAT-BN is designed to be a personally and emotionally significant intervention in which patients share important moments from their day-to-day lives in an effort to identify factors that contribute to BN episodes and discover strategies for change. The ICAT-BN skill set and accompanying skill cards do not replace the emotion-focused aspect of treatment, the value of the therapeutic relationship, and the personal struggle to make significant change. Rather, the skill cards and handouts are intended to extend and focus the treatment for the patient. It is imperative that the clinician understand that teaching the ICAT-BN skills and encouraging patients to practice them does not by itself constitute ICAT-BN therapy.

The Therapeutic Relationship in ICAT-BN

One of the most robust findings in the psychotherapy research literature is that regardless of the therapy modality, a strong therapeutic alliance fosters better outcome (Flückiger, Del Re, Wampold, Symonds, & Horvath, 2012; Horvath, 2000; Lambert, 2004). Typically, *therapeutic alliance* refers to shared goals between the patient and clinician, acceptance of the task that each needs to perform in the treatment, and an attachment bond between the patient and clinician (Bordin, 1979). Interestingly, there is mixed evidence regarding the importance of the therapeutic alliance in the treatment of BN. While some studies have suggested that a strong therapeutic alliance is associated with more positive outcomes in BN treatment (Constantino, Arnow, Blasey, & Agras, 2005; Treasure et al., 1999), other studies have failed to find that treatment alliance is associated with favorable clinical outcomes (e.g., Brown, Mountford, Waller, 2013; Loeb et al., 2005). While the evidence regarding the importance of therapeutic alliance in structured treatments for BN remains unclear, ICAT-BN is based on the fundamental principle that collaborative engagement in the treatment is clinically significant and that therapeutic alliance may facilitate such engagement.

The creation of a strong therapeutic alliance can be a difficult task and requires the clinician to be facile at building relationships with clients with BN, who often have difficulty with relationships (Constantino & Smith-Hansen, 2008). Both the clinician and the patient play a significant role in the development of their therapeutic

TABLE 4.2. Patient and Clinician Factors That Influence Outcome

Patient factors	Clinician factors
• Positive expectation of help and hope • Endorsement of the therapy rationale • Willingness to learn and to complete homework • Confidence in clinician • Ability to tolerate negative emotions • Engagement in self-disclosure • Commitment to the treatment	• Clinician well-being • Congruence between verbal and nonverbal aspects of clinician's speech • Use of interventions that elicit emotion • Tailoring the level of directness to the patient's level of resistance • Willingness to negotiate the tasks and goals of treatment • Modeling open and honest in-session communication • Eliciting unexpressed feelings about treatment and the patient's perception of the therapeutic process • Effective management of a patient's hostile process

relationship, and therefore the contributions of each should be examined. Empirical studies have identified a number of patient and clinician factors that affect psychotherapy alliance and outcomes (see Table 4.2). Some of these factors are more amenable to change than others (e.g., a sense of hope is easier to create than significant personality change). Factors particularly likely to influence outcome include clinician efforts to *engage* the patient thoroughly in the idea that he or she can be helped and that this treatment and this clinician can be effective. In addition, the patient's willingness to complete homework and understanding that treatment can at times be distressing may improve the likelihood of a positive treatment outcome (Clarkin & Levy, 2004).

Clinician factors also play an important role in enhancing outcome. Clinician skills and techniques in eliciting emotion and responding appropriately to the patient's noncollaborative behavior, particularly around areas of ambivalence or resistance to treatment, are important. Motivational interviewing (MI) techniques are particularly helpful here, as described in more detail in Chapter 5. Furthermore, being able to set goals in a flexible fashion and manage subtle forms of hostility are crucial (Beutler et al., 2004; Hill & Knox, 2009). Management of a disruption in the collaborative relationship between the clinician and patient (i.e., alliance rupture) will be discussed more thoroughly later in this chapter.

Therapeutic Collaboration Modes in ICAT-BN

The therapeutic relationship in ICAT-BN is *ideally* honest, supportive of the patient's adaptive functioning, highly collaborative, and sensitive to the patient's emotional states over the course of treatment. The therapeutic relationship may differ over the phases of ICAT-BN. For example, the clinician may be more oriented toward teaching and education as the patient attempts to implement the CARE plan and learn skills early on; whereas, in other phases of the treatment, the clinician may be less directly instructional and more likely to explore the patient's emotional experience inside and outside of therapy.

Ideally, the ICAT-BN clinician should be curious and interested in the patient's experience, adept in the technical aspects of ICAT-BN, and willing to explore emotionally difficult facets of the patient's life (particularly emotional states that appear to be associated with bulimic behavior or interfere with the patient's active collaboration in treatment). ICAT-BN clinicians are attentive to those aspects of the treatment that the patient wishes to avoid and address such avoidance in a collaborative fashion.

Figure 4.1 depicts four modes of the therapeutic relationship that support collaboration. First is the empathic mode, which refers to a variety of interventions designed to validate the patient's experience and truly understand their subjective world—for example:

"It sounds like being criticized by your coach was very painful for you. Can talk more about how it felt?"

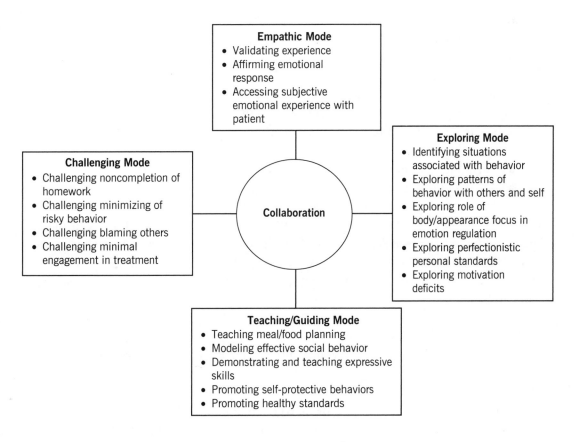

FIGURE 4.1. Therapeutic modes in ICAT.

The second is the exploring mode, whereby the clinician and patient together examine possible factors or experiences that might help to account for the patient's bulimic behavior—for example:

> "From what you wrote on your SEA Change Diary yesterday, it looks like the strong emotions you were having at the end of the day at work might have been linked with the binge episode you had in the car on your way home. Can we think about that possibility together?"

Third is a teaching mode, which refers to any time the clinician is directly trying to introduce new information to the patient. This is most clearly seen in Phase II during meal planning—for example:

> "Many years of research have helped us understand that skipping meals seems to contribute to binge eating. For that reason, it's really important to eat planned meals and snacks every few hours to help prevent binge-eating episodes."

Finally, the fourth mode is challenging. This mode is not a dramatic or hostile form of confrontation. Rather, it refers to raising awareness of certain behaviors that may be interfering with the treatment process—for example:

> "You seem a little distracted today, like your mind is somewhere else. It seems especially important for me to check in with you about it because it looks like you only completed a few self-monitoring forms this week."

Challenging may be appropriate when the patient is having difficulty completing homework, not truly participating in the treatment process, or has a response style that is not genuine in nature. Importantly, any of these modes may be utilized in an effort to establish a more collaborative relationship. Throughout treatment, the clinician remains sensitive to the ambivalence the patient may experience about change and thus validates and affirms the potential lack of collaboration as understandable; for example, the following statements reflect the clinician's awareness of such ambivalence:

> "You've helped me understand the powerful function that purging serves in helping you feel less upset when you end up in the middle of one of your parents' arguments."

> "Your mixed feelings about wanting to change make a lot of sense to me, and I appreciate your talking with me about your confusion so openly."

"The part I think you need to struggle with is your fear that you will gain weight if you quit purging, but your family and part of you want you to take that chance." Such interventions are essential in ICAT-BN because it is assumed that treatment is unlikely to be effective if a more collaborative stance is not established. Next, we offer more specific techniques for managing problematic therapeutic relationship issues in ICAT-BN.

Addressing Noncollaboration

ICAT-BN clinicians should always be vigilant for signs of noncollaboration, given that psychotherapy patients often express negative emotions about psychotherapy at some point during a course of treatment (Safran, Muran, Eubanks-Carter, 2011). In fact, it is often reasonable to discuss the likelihood of such noncollaborative episodes with the patient prospectively—for example:

"Our work in here requires that we let each other know when things don't feel right. Please let me know if I have said something that feels like I am not understanding or upsets you so that I can examine what I am doing and we can get back on track."

It may be helpful to discuss in advance the importance of shared goals and the necessity of correcting deviations from collaboration. This serves to normalize problems for patients and may help prevent them.

A clinician who suspects or detects evidence that the patient is not fully engaging in the treatment or appears ambivalent should share and discuss this observation with the patient. Of particular significance to ICAT-BN are the possible negative emotional responses the patient may have after trying to make adaptive changes in treatment. For example, if a Phase II patient is working on the CARE plan and the clinician notices frustration or incomplete meal planning, he or she may make a simple statement such as "I am wondering how this part of the treatment feels to you. Sometimes, patients find this part of the treatment difficult." Ideally, these types of comments will help to identify underlying feelings about the therapy. These emotions may be relatively simple, such as feeling frustrated about the difficulty of treatment, but may also be much more complex and intertwined with conceptions of the self (e.g., "I knew I could never do this, I am such a loser"). Often, simple clarification of underlying emotions and reassurance about expected rates of progress and anticipated difficulties will be sufficient to prompt the patient's further engagement and adherence to the treatment. Nonetheless, once the clinician notices ambivalence about the treatment, it is recommended that he or she periodically check in with patients about their emotional reactions to the treatment and how they believe they are doing.

While some patients will respond quite readily to simple clarification and encouragement, others will show a much more extensive and persistent ambivalence about treatment. Again, it is important to discuss this response with patients early and attempt to identify any difficulties they are having with treatment and their emotional reactions to these difficulties. If simple reassurance and redirection do not promote collaboration, the clinician should next review with the patient the nature of the collaborative working relationship in ICAT-BN. He or she should discuss with patients how he or she typically works with patients to try to understand the nature of the eating disorder symptoms they are experiencing, to appreciate the difficulty of change, and to introduce strategies and solutions throughout ICAT-BN that may help patients develop alternative ways of relating to themselves, other people, and food. The clinician may wish to emphasize that other models of caregiving in health care (e.g., dentistry or surgery) involve providers performing procedures *on* patients that lead to change and improved health. However, psychotherapy is a different health care technique, where it is not useful for the patient to passively wait to receive treatment delivered by a powerful clinician. Rather, a collaborative exchange model, such as that seen in teaching or coaching people to learn complex skills (e.g., musical instruments or sports), is more likely to be effective (Benjamin, 2003). This education and redirection will again help many patients return to a more productive and collaborative working relationship. However, there will remain a group of patients who are ambivalent about change and are highly unreliable in their engagement throughout treatment. MI techniques may have a limited effect on severely entrenched lack of collaboration. In such circumstances, the clinician may wish to attempt to identify the specifics of the interpersonal pattern that is being enacted between clinician and patient in the treatment (see Chapter 7). For example, the patient may display extreme hesitation to engage in the treatment, attempt to render the treatment ineffective, or have difficulty making the treatment a true priority. Such patterns are unlikely to promote change and should be addressed. In such situations it is not uncommon for clinicians to become too intensely focused upon creating change in the patient, and overzealous pursuit of change is unlikely to be effective. Regardless of the pattern or problem that is identified, the clinician attempts to return the treatment to a collaborative focus. As shown in the example below, noncollaboration can be approached directly with empathy and curiosity.

Example Dialogue

CLINICIAN: I noticed that you are still struggling with writing down what you are eating or planning to eat and also with bringing in situations that are difficult for you on the SEA Change Diaries. Can we talk about what filling out those forms is like for you?

PATIENT: Well, I don't really like filling out those forms, and I am really busy with work and school. I don't know.

CLINICIAN: Yeah, I get it. It sounds like you are a really busy person. But help me understand a little bit about your thoughts about treatment and how you are hoping to recover.

PATIENT: I am not sure what you mean.

CLINICIAN: I think it would be really helpful for me to try and understand something about how you're hoping treatment will work. You know, what you do, what I do, how the whole thing sort of comes together to help you recover.

PATIENT: Well, I don't really know. I guess I come here and I talk about my life and it makes me think about some things and then maybe I stop binge eating.

CLINICIAN: Yeah, often people think I might have something that I could do to them or for them which will make it happen, but it's probably good for us to get clear on that. I see it a little differently than you. Kind of more of a two-way street where you've got something you'd like to happen and I have an interest in trying to help you make that happen, but it really takes two of us to do it. We have to figure out how to really work together to make progress, which I am strongly interested in doing.

PATIENT: What do you exactly mean by work together? Am I doing this wrong?

CLINICIAN: No, you are not doing anything wrong. This is just hard work at times. Let's look at your question about what it means to work together. You know, like when I have a problem with my car, I just drop it off at the mechanic or if I have a bad tooth, I just go to the dentist and he sedates me and fixes the tooth. In either case, I don't have much to do; but in what we are trying to do, it doesn't seem to work that way. It requires you to really be engaged in our sessions and us working together. For me to really try and get what's going on with you, and work with you to find new ways of living your life. Then after we are done with each session, there is even more of a need for you to continue thinking about this out there in your daily life.

PATIENT: So is that why you want me writing things down and filling out these forms?

CLINICIAN: Exactly. After some days of not seeing each other, it's sort of a shorthand way for us to get back on track about the most important things that are happening in your life. That's why I like to see the Daily Food Records and the SEA Change Diaries.

PATIENT: Well, I suppose that makes sense, but I still don't like doing the forms.

CLINICIAN: Yes, I understand that and I appreciate your honesty about how you feel about doing them. But it remains a good way for us to work together, at least as I see it.

Therapeutic Impasses, Alliance Ruptures, and Alliance Repair

In addition to the emphasis on creating a therapeutic alliance, psychotherapy researchers have also focused on therapeutic impasses, alliance ruptures, and rupture repair. Therapeutic impasses are situations that occur during treatment and impede or stop clinical progress. The terms *therapeutic impasse* and *alliance rupture* are often used to describe the same phenomena in treatment. Safran, Muran, and Samstag (2002) define alliance ruptures as "tension or breakdown in the collaborative relationship between clinician and patient" (p. 236). Posttreatment interviews of successful and unsuccessful therapy cases demonstrate that impasses or ruptures are quite common in psychotherapy, and although a clinician can try to prevent them from occurring, they sometimes occur nonetheless. Psychotherapy patients report that they become angry or unhappy with their clinicians for a variety of reasons, such as the following: action or inaction by the clinician; perceived negative emotional reactions by the clinician; attempts by the clinician to decrease or control the patient's anger; a clinician encouraging the patient to be emotionally expressive but later distancing her- or himself because the patient is seen as demanding; or the clinician not responding to or ignoring the patient in some way (Hill & Knox, 2009). Luckily, repairing a rupture once it has occurred is not only possible, it can be helpful and initiate future positive change.

Therapeutic ruptures can be broadly described as falling into one of two categories: those characterized by withdrawal and those characterized by hostile confrontation (Hill & Knox, 2009; Safran & Muran, 2000). Different kinds of therapeutic acumen may be required to skillfully respond to these different types of ruptures. Clinicians often struggle with how best to respond when clients are hostile or directly confrontational (Hill & Knox, 2009). Such periods of complicated noncollaboration are best managed when the ICAT-BN clinician recognizes the problem and directly but sensitively discusses the pattern being enacted with the patient. Attempting to validate precipitants of the transaction and the clinician's role in the problem situation may help the patient to more effectively examine his or her behavior. The ultimate goal is to understand how the treatment was affected and agree to resume a more collaborative focus and continue the work. While hostile behavior toward the therapy or therapist is sometimes easy to perceive, recognizing when patients are withdrawing is not always straightforward. When withdrawal ruptures go unnoticed, they are more likely to remain unresolved. Unresolved ruptures can lead to premature termination of treatment. Many clients are quite hesitant to overtly express their dissatisfaction with the clinician. Therefore, how can a clinician detect when an alliance rupture has occurred if the patient does not bring it up directly? Psychotherapy researchers (Hill & Knox, 2009; Safran & Segal, 1996) suggest several key indicators that a rupture has occurred:

1. The patient indirectly communicates negative emotions about treatment through sarcasm.
2. The patient hints at perceived problems in the therapy by speaking about other relationships that have a similar interpersonal theme or pattern (e.g., the patient tells a story about how her father always told her she was wrong and then instructed her about the right way to think about things).
3. The patient disagrees with the clinician about the therapy goals.
4. The patient begins to passively submit or acquiesce to the all of the clinician's suggestions in a manner that suggests he or she is trying to avoid some conflict.
5. The patient does not collaborate with the clinician's attempt to work on some aspect of the patient's problem (thoughts, feelings, or behavior) because he or she believes the clinician has failed to understand the important function that the thought, feeling, or behavior has served.

Repairing a rupture requires clinicians to step back and observe the dyadic therapeutic process and become aware of their own feelings toward the patient and the action tendencies elicited by the patient before responding in order to avoid being drawn into the complementary response. For example, the "normal" human response to distrust or anger is hostility or defensiveness.

A number of empathic techniques have been developed and tested to help the clinician when these ruptures occur (Burns & Auerbach, 1996; Hill & Knox, 2009). Table 4.3 illustrates techniques that may be helpful with different kinds of impasses and alliance ruptures as well as clinician responses that may exacerbate these events. When clinicians are working through impasses or ruptures, their communication must have a genuinely respectful tone rather than a placating or sarcastic tone. Any hints of the latter will likely exacerbate the rupture.

SUMMARY

ICAT-BN places a significant emphasis on the quality of the therapeutic relationship and assumes that clinicians are technically competent and highly sensitive to the process of the treatment. The notion of a collaborative relationship between clinician and patient is paramount, and anytime the treatment does not seem to be collaborative, clear efforts should be made to redirect it into a more collaborative framework. Clinicians should be attentive to disturbances in the therapeutic relationship and address these directly and sensitively.

TABLE 4.3. Clinician's Helpful and Unhelpful Responses to Therapeutic Impasses or Alliance Ruptures

Helpful clinician responses	Generally unhelpful clinician responses
• Be aware of one's emotional reactions to the client.	• Responding defensively by arguing or disagreeing with the patient or by explaining or justifying one's actions.
• Identify the client's anger, listen carefully to the affect, and encourage elaboration of the anger.	• Allowing one's anxiety to impair empathic responding.
• Find the grain of truth in the patient's criticism even if it seems illogical or irrational (also called disarming).	• Making an insincere apology.
• Take some responsibility for the difficulty at hand and demonstrate that anger is possible in a good relationship.	• Ignoring the patient's expression of anger.
• Collaboratively explore the contribution of each person (patient and clinician) in creating this difficulty.	• Attributing the event that provoked the patient's anger to the patient's personality problems.
• Respond in an empathic manner with either thought empathy (paraphrasing what the patient said) or with feeling empathy (acknowledging how the patient is probably feeling). Check in with the patient to see if your guess about the patient's feelings is accurate.	• Interpreting the patient's current behavior toward the clinician as a re-creation of past dysfunctional relationships if the patient is not interpersonally or psychologically sophisticated.
• Use self-disclosure about the impact of the patient's communication (e.g., "I feel pulled to defend myself right now"). Use "I" rather than "you" to enhance the use of this technique. This communication must be used to serve the patient and not just to relieve the clinician.	• Pressuring the patient to respond or being overly directive.
• Make a sincere apology.	• Being overly supportive and too cautious or not being supportive enough and pushing the client too hard.
• Recognize and address a client's withdrawal by asking gentle and probing questions to draw out his or her thoughts and feelings.	• Failing to adapt one's conceptualization of the patient's problems or the function of those problems when the patient indicates it is incorrect.
• Raise the topic of unexpressed anger and explore any expressed affect.	
• Change the offending behavior if appropriate.	
• Affirm the patient's contributions in treatment.	
• Encourage the patient's continued active participation, seek the patient's feedback about therapy tasks, and negotiate new tasks if needed.	
• Express gratitude to the patient for discussing painful feelings honestly with you.	

Note. Based on Burns and Auerbach (1996, p. 153) and Hill and Knox (2009).

Part II

FOUR PHASES OF TREATMENT USING ICAT-BN

Chapter 5

Beginning, Engagement, and Education (Phase I)

Phase I of ICAT-BN attempts to promote engagement in treatment through two processes: (1) enhancing the therapeutic relationship and (2) introducing the treatment rationale and content through psychoeducation. Initially, the clinician attempts to enhance patient motivation using MI techniques. In addition, the clinician begins to educate the patient about emotions and their potential relevance to bulimic behavior. This process also includes providing psychoeducation about the importance of emotions more generally, as well as practicing emotional awareness both within and outside of sessions. Self-monitoring of behavior and emotion is also introduced in Phase I, which establishes a foundation for the more extensive self-monitoring and meal planning in Phase II.

MOTIVATIONAL INTERVIEWING

Phase I of ICAT-BN emphasizes MI in an effort to appreciate the patient's uncertainty about change and the emotional reactions that such change may elicit. This process is typically initiated in the first session by the clinician, who briefly reviews the history of the patient's bulimic symptoms and the individual and interpersonal context in which the behaviors now persist. This discussion helps the clinician understand the chronicity of the bulimic symptoms, assess the patient's self-concept over time, and begin to form hypotheses about the context in which these symptoms developed and are now maintained. These early clinical hypotheses regarding development and maintenance of these symptoms may or may not be confirmed over the course of treatment. The interpersonal and intrapersonal factors related to the bulimic symptoms will be an important focus of treatment in Phase III.

MI, developed by Miller and colleagues (e.g., Miller & Rollnick, 2002; Miller & Sovereign, 1989), is an approach first established for treatment of substance use disorders that focused on increasing the likelihood of a positive treatment outcome by enhancing the patient's motivation for change. Since that time, it has been applied more broadly to other types of psychopathology (Feinstein & Feinstein, 2004; Jones, Burckhardt, & Bennett, 2004; Moyers & Rollnick, 2004), including eating disorders (Vitousek, Watson, & Wilson, 1998; Treasure et al., 1999). MI, which focuses on the concept of ambivalence, is believed to be a particularly useful technique when working with patients who experience substantial conflict about the advantages and disadvantages of changing a behavior. Such ambivalence is commonly seen among individuals with bulimic symptoms, who are drawn to continue the behavior because of the perceived desirable consequences (e.g., regulating negative affect, controlling weight) while simultaneously wanting to stop the behavior because of its associated negative consequences (e.g., psychological distress, health risks, social and financial concerns). Because a clinician's emphasis on change risks increasing the patient's ambivalence, ICAT-BN focuses on addressing this conflict directly at the initial session with MI.

The content of MI in Phase I will be influenced, in part, by the nature of the treatment setting and assessment process. If a comprehensive assessment (see Berg & Peterson, 2013; Peterson, 2005) has already been conducted, the content of MI will focus on the patient's eating disorder history more generally. If the clinician is conducting the first session of ICAT-BN without a previous intake, the initial session can be extended to include more detailed questions about symptoms and history. In either case, the clinician should remain attuned to emotions and expressions of both ambivalence and motivation.

Notably, the use of MI techniques in ICAT-BN is not limited to sessions in Phase I. Rather, MI in ICAT-BN provides a framework the clinician maintains throughout treatment to address ambivalence about change whenever it occurs. As a result, ICAT-BN emphasizes the fundamental principles of MI throughout the course of treatment. These techniques include a consistent emphasis on empathy, ongoing discussion of the discrepancies between goals and outcomes, and an appreciation of the functional value of bulimic symptoms, as shown below.

Example Dialogue

PATIENT: I want to stop being bulimic, and that's why I decided to come to the clinic. But it's confusing, because sometimes I can't imagine ever stopping it.

CLINICIAN: It sounds like you have mixed feelings about changing. You want to stop, but it's hard to imagine not being bulimic.

PATIENT: Yes, exactly.

CLINICIAN: Can you talk some more about not being able to imagine stopping?

PATIENT: It's like I have been throwing up for so long that it's part of who I am. I throw up when I feel fat. I throw up when I am stressed about work. It's part of my routine.

CLINICIAN: If I am understanding what you are saying, being bulimic feels like it's part of your identity, and it can even make you feel better if you are feeling fat or stressed.

PATIENT: Right. But I don't like doing it, even if it's familiar.

CLINICIAN: What do you not like about doing it?

PATIENT: Well, honestly, it is gross. Sometimes when I am throwing up, I think about what I am doing and I feel completely disgusted.

CLINICIAN: It sounds like it's a dilemma for you. Being bulimic has some advantages. It feels familiar, it's part of your routine, and it can help you feel better sometimes when you are feeling fat or upset. But I also hear you saying that you don't like doing it and that it makes you feel disgusted. It makes me wonder how it fits in with your long-term goals. I mean, when we were talking about your life earlier, you described being very ambitious about your work. You also mentioned wanting to get married and traveling before you have kids. When you think about your future in that way, do you imagine being bulimic?

PATIENT: Honestly, no. I can't stand the thought of it.

CLINICIAN: So even though having bulimia has some advantages for you, it doesn't really fit in with how you imagine yourself in the future.

PATIENT: No, not at all. I think that's why I finally decided to get help.

The basic principle of MI centers on the reframing of treatment resistance as ambivalence. Through an empathic approach, the clinician aims to assist patients in developing a discrepancy between how they would like to be functioning and how they are actually functioning. Particularly important in ICAT-BN is focusing on how bulimic behaviors may contribute to this discrepancy. Crucially, the clinician initially aligns himself or herself with the potential advantages of not changing and expresses an explicit appreciation of the potential positive functions of the bulimic symptoms. In this context, the clinician only cautiously accepts the patient's expressed motivation for change. MI can be reintroduced throughout all phases of treatment at times of ambivalence.

The MI utilized in ICAT-BN can be summarized in five basic principles (Miller & Rollnick, 1991, 2002, 2012), which are described in detail in the next sections: express empathy, develop a discrepancy, avoid arguments, roll with resistance, and support self-efficacy.

Express Empathy

Empathy, in the context of MI in general and ICAT-BN in particular, can be conceptualized as an understanding of the patient's dilemma that is demonstrated through reflective listening. No effort is made to alter the patient's judgment directly; instead, the clinician focuses explicitly on gaining a comprehensive understanding of the ambivalence with the goal of reaching a judgment-free understanding of the patient's experience. Although Miller and Rollnick (1991) emphasize the importance of accepting the patient's ambivalence about treatment, they note that accepting the patient's view is different from agreeing with or approving of it (e.g., understanding the functions of the bulimic symptoms while believing that such behavior is nonetheless maladaptive). Through a collaborative, therapeutic interchange, the patient can gain an understanding that the clinician appreciates both sides of his or her ambivalence and the accompanying emotion. Notably, expressing empathy in the context of the patient's conflict can be quite disarming to the patient and can increase the patient's motivation for change as well as therapeutic rapport.

Develop a Discrepancy

In discussing the patient's motivation and hesitation about changing the bulimic behavior patterns, the clinician can strive to make this ambivalence explicit in the initial ICAT-BN sessions. Asking the patient to describe the full range of his or her feelings about the possibility of change, especially the potential functions and advantages of the bulimic symptoms, can be helpful in this process. In this context, discussions about future plans and objectives are also useful in setting up an explicit discrepancy between current behavior and long-term goals. Having the clinician "side" with reasons not to change can be especially powerful in this process. In ICAT-BN, it is especially important for the clinician to have the patient describe various aspects of the discrepancy while simultaneously attending to the associated emotional reactions. When successful, this process results in the patient beginning to develop a well-articulated motivation for change rather than the clinician attempting to convince the patient to change. This outcome is depicted in the transcript below.

Example Dialogue

CLINICIAN: In what ways have your binge-eating symptoms been helpful to you?

PATIENT: No one has ever asked me that before. Everyone just says how dangerous it is to be bulimic.

CLINICIAN: Actually, we do think it's very important to understand what might be positive for you about bingeing, especially when you are just starting treatment.

PATIENT: Well, I do get to eat whatever I want, and if I have had a bad day, bingeing makes me forget about whatever is upsetting me.

CLINICIAN: So having binges helps you feel less upset and makes you feel freer to eat what you want.

PATIENT: Yes, exactly. But there are problems, too, which is why I decided to get help.

CLINICIAN: Tell me about those.

PATIENT: Well, it's like I have this secret life. I eat in secret. None of my family or friends knows. I feel like I am living a lie, which is awful.

CLINICIAN: So the dishonesty feels bad to you.

PATIENT: Yes. And I feel really sick after I binge. Also, I am obsessed with food. All I ever think about is what I've eaten, what I shouldn't eat, and what I'm going to eat. It's hard to concentrate on anything else.

CLINICIAN: What other things do you wish you could concentrate on instead of thinking about food?

PATIENT: Well, like when my friends are talking. And also my music. Being a musician is really important to me, and sometimes it's hard to focus on it because I'm bingeing or obsessing with food.

CLINICIAN: So when you think of your life 5 years from now, what do you hope it will be like?

PATIENT: I think about having a successful music career, close friends, travel, and stuff like that.

CLINICIAN: Where does the bulimia fit in?

PATIENT: It doesn't.

CLINICIAN: So if I am understanding you correctly, I hear there is a real split for you here. On one hand, the binge eating helps soothe you when you are upset. But the binge eating makes it hard to concentrate on things you care about, it takes a lot of time away from other things you value, it makes you feel sick, and it causes you to feel badly about yourself for being dishonest. And, I'm struck by the fact that when you think about the future and the life you want to be leading, there is really no room for the binge eating and you really don't want to be dealing with it.

PATIENT: Yes, that's right.

Avoid Arguments

In ICAT-BN, every effort is made to avoid marked confrontation and argument with the patient. If resistance occurs in the form of argumentation or debate, the clinician should try a different avenue or approach to address the motivational conflict at hand rather than escalating the confrontation.

Roll with Resistance

The alternative to struggling against the patient's resistance is using it to one's advantage. Rolling with resistance is done by reframing the resistance as understandable from the patient's perspective, and offering new perceptions, views, or approaches to the patient. Again, these perspectives are not forced upon the patient but are offered as options or alternatives that the patient is free to accept or reject, as illustrated in the dialogue example below.

Example Dialogue

CLINICIAN: We generally find that when patients can consume three meals and one or two snacks a day, it helps them to reduce their binge eating.

PATIENT: There is no way I could do that. I would quit treatment.

CLINICIAN: I imagine that the idea of eating meals is not only foreign to you, but also might be scary. What do you think might happen?

PATIENT: I'd just lose it. I'd get fat.

CLINICIAN: Yeah, maybe one of the benefits of your eating patterns has been to give you an escape from negative thoughts about your appearance. Are there other ways your current eating behavior might have helped you?

This topic may lead to a discussion of other perceived benefits of the bulimic behavior, and the clinician follows this discussion rather than trying to emphasize the importance of following a meal plan.

Support Self-Efficacy

Inherent in the MI approach are two key ideas: first, the belief that the patient's behavior can change; second, the belief that the patient will play a crucial role in making this change. Thus, substantial emphasis is placed on forming a collaborative relationship that encourages and respects the patient's autonomy and avoids a controlling, authoritarian stance.

The Collaborative Treatment Relationship during MI

Avoiding arguments with the patient and rolling with resistance, both tenets of MI, are important principles that should guide the clinician in most cases. Such a strategy, coupled with the patient's wish to change (although perhaps ambivalent), frequently directs treatment in a productive direction. However, there will be occasions where some patients show a profound disengagement from treatment and are simply not contributing to a collaborative transaction with the clinician. Clarifying and understanding their ambivalence is obviously important in such circumstances, but the therapeutic modality of challenging, outlined in Chapter 4, may also need to be introduced in extreme cases of disengagement and lack of progress. Especially in short-term treatments (e.g., 21 sessions) a more direct examination of the patient's lack of collaboration may be required to gain some understanding of therapeutic impasses and stalemates. Consequently, if a clinician does not see some degree of patient engagement in the process, she or he should initially approach this problem from an MI perspective, but in the absence of progress, a more direct therapeutic challenge that emphasizes the importance of collaboration may be indicated.

INTRODUCING THE ICAT-BN MODEL

Early in Phase I, typically in the first session, the clinician provides Handout 5.1, "Understanding Bulimia Nervosa." This handout describes the circumstances leading up to bulimic symptoms according to the ICAT-BN model. It may be useful to walk the patient through the graphic of the model shown in Handout 5.1[1] before providing the handout that describes the model more fully. The clinician can emphasize that aspects of the model may or may not be relevant to the patient's own experience. In the first session, Handout 5.2, "Overview of Treatment," can be given along with Handout 5.3, "Preparing for Treatment." The latter is a questionnaire that the clinician can suggest the patient complete as homework and bring to the following session for discussion with the clinician. These handouts are useful for increasing motivation for change and determining the patient's readiness to work on eating disorder behaviors. Clinicians should note when homework is assigned and make sure to ask about the assignment in the next session.

INTRODUCTION OF EMOTIONS

As early as possible in ICAT-BN, the clinician will begin to introduce the significance of emotions. While there are many models of emotion, in ICAT-BN clinicians teach patients that there are six primary emotions: joy, sadness, fear, anger, disgust, and surprise (Ekman & Friesen, 2003). Other important emotions to discuss may include contempt, guilt, anxiety, confusion, and shame. ICAT-BN clinicians

---

[1] See Part III, pages 159–219, for all handouts.

communicate to their patients that emotions are an essential part of being human: negative emotions cannot be avoided and positive emotions can be fully experienced. Some patients with BN often feel overwhelmed by and may have difficulty coping with and tolerating their painful emotions, while other patients may have difficulty identifying or describing their emotional experience.

A key focus in ICAT-BN is helping patients experience and understand their emotions, especially any negative emotions that precede bulimic behaviors. Negative emotions appear to increase the likelihood of eating-related urges in some individuals (Agras & Telch, 1998), and bulimic behaviors help patients to manage their strong emotions albeit in a maladaptive manner (Smyth et al., 2007). An important step in this process is to ensure patients can identify their emotions. In order to teach patients to identify their emotions, clinicians encourage them to notice their physical sensations, facial expressions, and the actions they feel motivated to take in response to the emotions. A key goal in ICAT-BN is to help patients make healthy behavioral choices in spite of their emotional experiences. Identifying the action urges associated with negative emotions is important in disrupting the link between negative emotions and subsequent bulimic behaviors.

Handout 5.1 may be helpful in illustrating the importance of emotions in maintaining bulimic symptoms. The following aspects of emotions are emphasized to patients in the early sessions of ICAT-BN.

1. Emotions are an important and normal part of experience that help us understand that something important is occurring. Emotions prepare us to take action. Usually, having an emotion lets us know that there is something that we need and the emotion motivates us to act to help meet our need. In addition, behaviors and urges may be helpful in identifying specific emotions as well as situations that may trigger them, a concept that is emphasized in Phase III.

2. Some actions may provide short-term relief from negative emotions and temporarily meet our needs, but they can also produce problems. For example, avoiding a difficult problem situation may provide initial relief, but avoidance does not solve the problem. Also, ruminating about a problem, such as not living up to a standard, may also provide a temporary distraction from the actual immediate negative feeling but ultimately increase the negative emotional state. Emotions can be set off by a variety of different events or situations. A person may not be consciously aware of what is triggering these feelings, and gaining such awareness may be useful.

3. Emotions are experienced as sensations in both the mind and body. We can use bodily sensations in our head, stomach, and muscles to help determine when we are experiencing emotions. Often, these experiences can be difficult to identify. Handout 5.4, "Beginning to Notice My Feelings," provides pictures of faces with

examples of different types of emotions; they can be particularly helpful for individuals who have difficulty labeling their emotional experience. As illustrated by Handout 5.4, specific emotions are linked with specific facial expressions. The clinician can use this handout in session whenever a patient struggles with identifying an emotion as well as encouraging the patient to refer to the handout between sessions to practice labeling emotions. These faces serve as an emotional "dictionary" and can help the patient develop a more nuanced emotional vocabulary. Together with the clinician, the patient can examine different types of emotions in order to practice identifying and labeling his or her own feelings.

INTRODUCTION OF THE FEEL SKILL

A critical component of Phase I is the introduction of the first core skill, the FEEL skill. It is designed to increase the patient's awareness, identification, and experiencing of emotions. The skill is introduced in the first and second sessions using Handout 5.5, and the clinician underscores the importance of this skill throughout treatment.

When introducing the FEEL skill, the clinician can emphasize that bulimic behavior may serve as a means of regulating emotional states. Learning to be aware of these states and their precipitants, and finding alternative ways to manage them, can enhance the chances for behavioral change. The clinician can also emphasize that people are often unaware of emotions as they are occurring and that increasing efforts to be aware of emotional states can be helpful. Furthermore, it is important to try to label emotional experiences. Treatment is directed toward trying to help the client identify meaningful labels for his or her experiences and then discuss them in therapy.

As shown in Handout 5.5, the FEEL skill consists of four steps:

1. Focus by finding a quiet place to sit and notice body sensations.
2. Experience emotion by allowing a feeling to come and noticing any other accompanying emotions.
3. Examine the strongest feeling as well as where that feeling might be coming from or what is behind the feeling.
4. Label it or give it a name.

Handout 5.5 should be given to patients when the clinician introduces this skill. The following clinical example illustrates how the clinician can provide education about emotion early in Phase I.

Example Dialogue

CLINICIAN: In this treatment, we believe that emotions are linked to bulimic behavior and that often people who struggle with binge eating and purging are not aware of their emotions. Because feelings are such a normal part of life, we think it is important to be aware of them, understand them, and express them, particularly in therapy. If you are willing, I would be very interested in knowing about your emotional experiences and, in fact, we have a specific skill in this treatment designed to help with that.

PATIENT: Um . . . honestly, I think that could be hard for me.

CLINICIAN: Tell me more . . . what might make it hard?

PATIENT: Well, I try *not* to focus on feelings. I don't like it. One of the reasons I have three jobs is so that I don't have time to stop and think about whatever is upsetting me.

CLINICIAN: I really appreciate that you are aware of how hard that might be for you. It also suggests that we might want to start using the FEEL skill to identify your feelings very gradually—maybe spending just a few minutes at a time sitting with how you are feeling.

PATIENT: Like 30 minutes?

CLINICIAN: I was thinking more like 5 minutes at the start . . . just following the steps for the FEEL skill to see what it's like. We find that the more you practice it, the easier it gets. Would you be willing to try it?

PATIENT: Yeah, I think I could do 5 minutes at a time, but I am not sure that I'll be able to figure out what I'm actually feeling.

CLINICIAN: It's great that you are willing to try it. We have a handout [Handout 5.4] that might be helpful in figuring out what you are feeling.

At this point, the clinician can continue to emphasize the specific elements of the FEEL skill and work with the patient to find ways in which the skill can be practiced on a regular basis. The FEEL skill will be practiced in session, including during the session when the skill is introduced, and patients are encouraged to use it outside of sessions throughout the course of ICAT-BN. As part of developing the FEEL skill, the clinician must remain focused on the patient's emotional reactions within each session. This emotion-focused aspect of the treatment is essential in assisting the patient to identify feelings as they occur and begin to cope effectively with emotional experiences. The clinician is encouraged to acknowledge and explore patients' feelings as they occur in the session, including asking questions (e.g., "Can you describe what the feeling is like for you as you consider change?"). This query may then be followed by a series of questions or statements that deepen or clarify the emotional response (e.g., "What seems most concerning to you?"; "What are you noticing in your body?"). By exploring emotions that occur in the session, the clinician helps set the tone of the treatment's emphasis on emotion early in treatment.

SELF-MONITORING FOOD INTAKE AND EMOTIONS

At the end of Session 1 or during Session 2, the clinician introduces the patient to self-monitoring using Handout 5.7, "Daily Food Record," and Handout 5.8, "Sample Completed Daily Food Record" (Figure 5.1 also shows an example of a completed form.) The clinician can describe the rationale for self-monitoring in detail (as well as providing Handout 5.6, "Why Write Down What You Eat?"). For example, the clinician can explain that the self-monitoring process is thought to be critical in facilitating changes in bulimic behaviors because it provides detailed data for discussion during therapy sessions and facilitates self-awareness and an understanding of symptom patterns and precipitants. In addition, these records provide valuable information to the patient and the clinician about emotions and their link to binge eating and bulimic symptoms, particularly "momentary" data. The clinician can also inform patients that writing down what they eat, by itself, has been found to lead to reductions in binge eating and other behaviors that accompany an eating disorder (Agras, Schneider, Arnow, Raeburn, & Telch, 1989). Some patients may have completed food logs in the past and found the process to be aversive (especially in the context of formal weight-loss programs). The clinician can emphasize that self-monitoring will be used differently in ICAT-BN, and that the purpose is for the patient and clinician to collaborate on finding what is most helpful for recovery. The momentary focus of treatment can also be emphasized in the context of self-monitoring and the importance of "in the moment" data. Clinicians may want to mention that one study revealed when patients were interviewed after completion of a cognitive-behavioral treatment, they reported that although they did not enjoy completing food logs at the beginning of therapy, they realized by the end of treatment that it was one of the most helpful aspects of the program (Mussell et al., 1997). In addition, the clinician should be direct in stating that the food records will not be judged or criticized, but that these records are an important part of the therapeutic collaboration as well as a way to monitor change. Most patients are highly self-conscious about sharing detailed information about their eating patterns, particularly their binge-eating episodes. However, as the clinician reacts with acceptance, curiosity, and interest during self-monitoring reviews in subsequent sessions, most patients become increasingly comfortable with the process. In addition, reviewing self-monitoring data collaboratively can help develop therapeutic rapport and deepen engagement early in treatment. The following points can be emphasized in introducing self-monitoring:

Daily Food Record

Date _____

Time	Type* (M, S, R, V, L, D, E, B)	Food/Beverage	Notes (location, feelings)
7:00	M, R	½ bagel, plain Water (1 bottle)	Breakfast at home Feeling fat, trying to cut back
10:00		Coffee (1 cup)	Work, stressed about meeting
12:00	M, R	Salad (2 cups) Water (1 bottle)	At work, preparing for meeting; Feeling worried about meeting; Trying not to eat much, skipped salad dressing
2:30	S, R	Nonfat yogurt (1/2 cup)	Worried about meeting; Saw cookies in the break room; Had yogurt instead of cookies
3:00	S	2 cookies (chocolate chip)	Ate during meeting; Unhappy about meeting; Mad at myself for not doing a better presentation
3:30	B	5 cookies (chocolate chip)	Can't stop eating; mad, sad
5:30	B	3 cheeseburgers; Fries (5 cups); Milkshake (1 large)	Stopped at drive-through; Eating out of control; Upset but can't stop; Have to purge, scared of weight
5:45	V		Stopped at store; might as well keep eating; feel disgusted with myself; feel fat
6:00	B	Cookies (sandwich), 1 pkg; Ice cream, (2 pints)	
6:30	V		Feel gross, sad, mad
9:00		Water (1 bottle)	Tired, going to bed
Exercise (Type, Duration):		None	

*Type: M = meal; S = snack; R = restricting; V = vomiting; L= laxative; D= diuretic; E = exercise; B = binge/overeating/eating more than planned/loss of control.

FIGURE 5.1. Example of a completed Daily Food Record.

1. Patients should write down everything they eat and drink (with the exception of small amounts of water) as soon as possible after it has been consumed in order to increase self-awareness and accuracy. For this reason, they need to be able to access their food record at all times. Part of the session may need to be devoted to the logistics of where to keep the food record so that it is accessible.

2. Some patients may complain that writing down their food intake makes them more preoccupied with eating, shape, and weight. They can be reassured that this increase in problematic preoccupations is usually temporary and subsides once self-monitoring becomes a habit (Fairburn, 2008); however, one of the primary goals of self-monitoring is to increase self-awareness of eating (as well as emotions) on a permanent basis in order to reduce bulimic symptoms.

3. Considerable time should be spent in Phase I introducing the food record and reviewing a sample food record. During the session in which monitoring is introduced, it is helpful to label a blank log for that day and to have patients write what they have already eaten that day (although emphasize that typically they will be writing down what they ate immediately). The clinician should provide the patient with plenty of blank self-monitoring forms, including extras in case the subsequent session is rescheduled.

4. The version of the food record given at Session 2 does not include a place to note whether the food eaten was on the patient's plan, which is added in the CARE skill in Phase II. Once the CARE skill and plan are introduced in Phase II, the CARE form should be used for self-monitoring instead of the version introduced in Phase I.

TRANSITIONING FROM PHASE I TO PHASE II

Typically, after one to three sessions of Phase I, patients are clearly ready to move on to Phase II. In spite of some degree of ambivalence and uncertainty, they make clear statements that they wish to make changes in their eating behavior and make an effort toward recovery. Indications of readiness can be seen in declarative statements of intent and motivation (e.g., "I am ready to try"; "I need to do this"). In cases wherein there is an extreme ambivalence and reluctance to move ahead, we would recommend that clinicians thoroughly examine the ambivalence but recommend moving into Phase II as an experiment. Patients should be informed that Phase II will be focused on modifying eating behavior and directly addressing urges for bulimic behavior, but that this phase can be approached gradually by establishing small and strategic goals. In the randomized controlled trial and the pilot studies testing ICAT-BN, there were no instances of patients dropping out at this point in the treatment.

SUMMARY

Phase I focuses on introducing ICAT-BN in the context of MI and an emphasis on the importance of emotional awareness. This phase also provides the foundation of self-monitoring, which is introduced early in treatment and is continued in various formats. MI is also useful in developing therapeutic rapport and, although it is emphasized early in Phase I, it can be utilized throughout treatment.

Chapter 6

Making Plans for Eating and Managing Urges (Phase II)

The primary goals of Phase II are to facilitate changes in eating patterns through emotional self-awareness and the development of adaptive coping skills. Because Phase I of ICAT-BN is typically brief and consists of only one or two sessions, the shift to Phase II often builds from the content of MI, with the patient stating an explicit interest (with or without ambivalence) in changing eating patterns and bulimic behaviors. Because Phase II involves significant behavioral change in the planned consumption of meals and snacks, the focus on emotional experience both within and outside of sessions is especially important during this phase. The initial Phase II sessions focus on continuing to review self-monitoring of food intake and emotions, as well as practicing the FEEL skill. In addition, the clinician works collaboratively to help the patient understand the link between momentary emotions and bulimic symptoms. The clinician introduces the rationale for meal planning through in-session discussion and psychoeducation provided in the handouts.

Typically, Phase II starts at Session 3 (or, for highly motivated patients, Session 2) following the introductory sessions of Phase I and lasts for approximately six sessions (e.g., Sessions 3–8). At the initiation of Phase II, patients are typically familiar with the FEEL skill and self-monitoring procedures. In the initial session of Phase II (e.g., Session 3), the clinician begins to provide the rationale for eating planned meals and snacks in the context of self-monitoring reviews and psychoeducational discussions including handouts. In introducing the CARE (Calmly Arrange Regular Eating) skill, typically around Session 4 or 5, the clinician works with the patient to establish meal plans with a particular emphasis on understanding emotions that arise with this shift in eating patterns. The middle sessions of Phase II (e.g., Sessions 5, 6, and 7) typically focus on implementing and reviewing the patient's experience with meal planning. In addition, adaptive coping using the ACT (Adaptive Coping Technique) skill is emphasized to help the patient with urge management. The GOAL (Goals and Objectives Affect Life-Moments) skill is also introduced during Phase II to facilitate short-term goal setting in the context of treatment. Throughout Phase II and particularly toward its end (i.e., Sessions 7–9), Phase III concepts may be discussed as examples relevant to that phase are reported on self-monitoring forms. These include the role of interpersonal experiences, self-evaluation, and self-regulation behaviors in eliciting momentary emotions. However, Phase II typically remains focused on supporting changes in eating behavior and identifying precipitants of emotion dysregulation not addressed in depth until Phase III. The clinician's monitoring of Phase III concepts during Phase II facilitates the transition between Phases II and III.

INITIAL PHASE II SESSIONS

The transition from Phase I to Phase II can be bridged by the ongoing self-monitoring of eating patterns and emotions introduced in Phase I (see Handout 5.7 and Figure 5.1). The early sessions in Phase II (typically Sessions 3–6) include in-session reviews of self-monitoring forms with an emphasis on the link between eating behaviors and emotions that occurs prior to and following any type of food consumption or bulimic symptoms. Focusing on emotion is important when self-monitoring forms include a description of feelings (especially in the context of bulimic symptoms) and when any emotions (e.g., sadness, anxiety) are described or observed in session.

Example Dialogue

CLINICIAN: So can you talk me through your self-monitoring form [Handout 5.7] from yesterday in more detail? From what I am seeing on your form, it looks like you had a lot going on last night.

PATIENT: Yes. So as I wrote here, I had dinner with my parents at their house, and my brother was there too. I had planned to just have a salad and maybe a little barbeque chicken because my father was grilling. I didn't want to stay at their house too long because I wanted to get back to my dorm to finish homework. So I got there and we watched the end of the football game together. I was kind of bored and ended up eating some chips during the game, which made me feel fat and bad about my lack of self-control and I decided to eat even less at dinner. We sat down to dinner and I took a little salad and started to eat. Then, my parents started asking me a bunch of questions about my grades at college—like what scores I had gotten on my tests so far, whether I am going to get A's in my classes, and stuff like that.

I tried to answer all of their questions and even though my grades are good so far, I started to feel worse and worse as they were asking me questions. (*Eyes fill with tears.*)

CLINICIAN: If you don't mind my interrupting you, I notice that you are getting tearful. Can you tell me how you are feeling right now, as we are talking?

PATIENT: Well, talking about it gets me upset all over again. I feel like no matter what I do, they always ask me so many questions like they are waiting for me to mess up my grades in college. When I am at school and studying, I feel okay. But when my parents start asking me about school, I get upset and insecure. (*Continues to cry.*)

CLINICIAN: I can see how upset you are. Can you describe for me what you are experiencing right at this moment?

PATIENT: My stomach is in knots, and I just feel so sad—like I always disappoint my parents no matter how hard I try to do well and I just want to cry.

CLINICIAN: Yes, I understand. And I really appreciate your describing your emotions to me—your sadness, the knots in your stomach. Can you tell me more about how you are feeling right now?

PATIENT: It's a feeling right behind my eyes—like I can't control the tears.

CLINICIAN: What's it like for you to sit with these feelings with me? Do you feel like you should be controlling your tears?

PATIENT: It's funny, because on my way to meet with you today, I figured that I would just mention last night without talking too much about it because I was afraid to get upset. I mean, I have only met with you a few times and here I am just falling apart. But now that I am actually crying, it's not as embarrassing as I thought it would be. I feel really sad as we are talking but sort of calm too—like talking about it makes the whole thing last night seem a little better, and I am not sure why I was so worried about getting upset in front of you.

CLINICIAN: It takes a lot of courage to be so honest with me—not just talking about your feelings, but showing me how upset you are. It sounds like it's less embarrassing than you thought it would be and might even be helping you feel less upset. Is the sadness that you are feeling now similar to how you felt last night with your parents?

PATIENT: Yes, exactly. Well, last night I was sad and also worried. I started to feel like maybe I didn't know what I was doing in college, that maybe I would mess up on the math test I had on Monday morning. I felt super stressed and the next thing I know I was sitting at dinner and started eating bread with butter, and then potatoes, and even dessert. I was answering my parents' questions and eating at the same time, just counting the minutes until I could leave. Then I got into my car and drove to the gas station, ate a bunch more food that I bought, and purged behind the building. By the time I got back to my dorm, my throat hurt and I felt kind of spacey. I ended up going to bed early and then getting up this morning to study for my math test.

As this example illustrates, the clinician immediately focused on the in-session emotions as they emerged in discussing the patient's self-monitoring. The clinician provided validation and support as well as examining how the patient experienced sharing these feelings in session. The clinician also helped the patient identify the physical manifestations of these feelings and, after a thorough discussion, guided the discussion back to the example from the self-monitoring form. In the case material below, the clinician continues to use the example from the self-monitoring form to illustrate the importance of momentary emotion in eliciting bulimic symptoms.

Example Dialogue

CLINICIAN: So it sounds like you had initially planned to limit what you ate while you were at your parents' but ended up eating a little during the football game, felt worse about yourself, and then decided to restrict even more than you had planned during dinner.

PATIENT: Yes, exactly.

CLINICIAN: From what you described, and I see what you wrote on your form, feeling bored seemed to be linked to eating the chips.

PATIENT: Yes. I mean, everyone was watching the game, but I wasn't really into it and I was bored. The chips looked really good and they were right there, so I ended up eating them and I felt fat and disgusted with myself because I had planned to not each much at all.

CLINICIAN: It's helpful for us to learn together that feeling bored was linked to eating more than you had planned, or that eating was even a distraction.

PATIENT: Yes, it was a distraction, but then I felt worse.

CLINICIAN: Yes, as you were saying, the eating made you feel worse about yourself and then you felt more upset.

PATIENT: Yes, like I had failed in my self-control. And then when my parents started to ask me all those questions about my grades, it felt like I had failed in their eyes too and then I got even more upset.

CLINICIAN: Yes, feeling like you didn't live up to your own standards and maybe your parents' standards too made you feel sad and worried, as you described earlier. Then what happened with the eating as you felt those emotions at dinner?

PATIENT: I felt like I had eaten too much already because of the chips, I felt like maybe I was failing at school and my parents were disappointed, and then I saw the bread and just really wanted to eat it. I try not to eat refined carbohydrates and it was white bread, not wheat bread, but then I just ate it. And then I figured that if I was eating bread and blowing it anyway, I might as well put butter on it. It tasted really good and even though I was upset about what my parents were saying, it was like I could just eat whatever I wanted. And then I couldn't stop eating, and I was kind of upset but sort of numb all at the same time. On the way home, I figured I might as well eat more food that I would never eat if I weren't going to throw up, so I bought a bunch of cookies and ate those, then threw up. By the time I got back to my dorm, I was completely exhausted and just went to sleep.

CLINICIAN: You are really helping me understand how closely linked your eating was last night with your feelings. First, you ate the chips when you were bored and then you ate the bread and butter at dinner when you were feeling so sad and worried. It almost seems like the eating might have helped in the moment when you were so upset.

PATIENT: I mean, I hate bingeing because I feel so disgusting, but honestly it did help me get through dinner and just kept me focused on something until I could leave. And then I was planning what else I could buy and eat on the way back to my dorm.

CLINICIAN: I think understanding how the eating can actually serve a function for you—that it might help you feel the emotions less intensely, to distract you from feeling so upset—might be really important for us to discuss.

PATIENT: Yes. And if I hadn't binged and thrown up, I would have just lay in bed thinking about dinner over and over in my mind. It was terrible that I didn't study for my test last night but at least I could just go to sleep.

CLINICIAN: It sounds like the bingeing and purging might have been useful for you in trying to manage your feelings when you were upset. It also sounds like it was a relief to eat the bread and butter and be free from your own strict standards about what you can and can't eat.

PATIENT: I mean, I shouldn't be eating bread and butter. I just shouldn't. But sometimes I just get so tired of thinking about every single thing I eat.

CLINICIAN: It sounds like that might be especially true when you are upset about something.

PATIENT: Yes, I think that's true.

CLINICIAN: And we will also start to focus on the fact that you certainly *can* eat bread and butter—especially in a planful way when you aren't at risk of a binge.

In this example, the clinician helped the patient identify the momentary emotions that were linked with her eating patterns as well as the potential functions of her bulimic symptoms in trying to regulate her feelings. Although the clinician did not describe the concepts in detail, high self-standards and excessive self-control were mentioned as precipitants of negative emotion that might be useful to focus on during Phase III sessions. Throughout this example, the clinician provided validation and guidance toward understanding the link between emotions and eating patterns. In addition, the clinician aimed to deepen the patient's ability to identify and tolerate emotions as well as providing information about eating high-risk foods in a planned manner.

ADDITIONAL GUIDELINES
FOR SELF-MONITORING DISCUSSIONS

Ideally, the in-session review of self-monitoring forms in the early stage of Phase II is a collaborative process between the patient and the clinician. The patient can be encouraged to take the lead in talking through the forms with the clinician, who can use questions to guide the discussion. Ideally, the clinician can make duplicate copies of the self-monitoring forms when the patient arrives in order to read the content that the patient describes during the review. In-session Phase II self-monitoring discussions typically emphasize the following content:

1. **Feelings or emotions that are described in the logs.** Asking about emotional content reinforces the importance of emotions, helps the patient develop the FEEL skill, and is useful in identifying potential links between emotions and eating patterns.

Example: "I notice here you wrote down that you were feeling mad at your husband yesterday morning. Can you tell me more about feeling mad?"

2. **Feelings that arise in the context of reviewing the self-monitoring logs.** As illustrated in the example at the beginning of this chapter, the clinician's attentiveness to facial expressions and body posture during the discussion of the self-monitoring logs (as well as throughout the entire session) is helpful in focusing on in-session emotions.

Example: "I notice that as we are discussing what happened at work yesterday, your face changed expressions; can you talk me through what you are feeling right at this moment?"

3. **Phase III core concepts.** Although self-regulatory style, interpersonal problems, and self-evaluation become a focus of treatment in Phase III, these concepts can be introduced if they arise during Phase II self-monitoring review.

Example: "As you were describing to me how badly you were feeling about your body shape yesterday, it made me wonder if some of your distress comes from having very high standards for yourself and feeling like you don't live up to them."

4. **Motivational issues that are noted on the self-monitoring form or arise in discussion.** The patient may continue to express ambivalence about change during discussions of self-monitoring. Discussing these feelings provides ideal opportunities for further motivational enhancement strategies introduced at Phase I.

Example: "I hear you describing how you rely on binge eating and purging to help you feel less anxious, and it almost sounds like you are having some mixed feelings about the prospect of giving it up. Perhaps we could talk some more about how bingeing and purging may be helpful to you and how you are feeling about the possibility of change?"

5. **Issues relevant to therapeutic rapport.** Patients are often hesitant to share detailed information about food they consume during binge-eating episodes because of shame or embarrassment, particularly when discussing self-monitoring content. Watching for indications of shame or fear in the written self-monitoring forms (e.g., sections that appear to be blank or incomplete) or during these discussions can be valuable for exploring emotions and deepening engagement.

Example: "I notice on your self-monitoring form that you wrote the word *binge* for Wednesday night's episode but didn't actually write down what you ate during the binge. Let's talk about what made it hard to write that down. Were you concerned about sharing it with me?"

BUILDING THE RATIONALE FOR MEAL PLANNING AND THE CARE SKILL

One of the most crucial components of Phase II occurs several sessions into this phase (e.g., sessions 4–6) when the clinician introduces the CARE (Calmly Arrange Regular Eating) skill to help the patient eat planned meals and snacks in order to interrupt his or her bulimic patterns. There are a number of reasons why meal planning is fundamental for recovery and especially important to introduce early in treatment. First, as described in Handout 6.1, "Why Eat Regular Meals and Snacks," adequate food intake is essential in alleviating the starvation-related nutritional and physiological conditions that often elicit binge-eating behavior (Keys, Brožek, Henschel, Mickelsen, & Taylor, 1950). The most valuable data on the effects of semi-starvation are from an investigation conducted by Ancel Keys and colleagues

(1950) near the end of World War II. The purpose of the study was to determine the best strategies to help prisoners of war recover from starvation by examining how they were affected by the nutritional composition of different foods and by vitamin supplementation provided to facilitate weight restoration. Study participants were healthy young adult male volunteers who were conscientious objectors and screened to ensure their mental and physical health. The participants were placed on calorically restricted diets in order to reduce their body weight to mimic the effects of semi-starvation. During this phase of the study, the participants began to experience many of the symptoms that patients with eating disorders (especially those engaging in significant dietary restriction) experience, including negative emotions (e.g., depression, anxiety, irritability), a loss of interest and pleasure in previously engaging activities, impaired concentration, preoccupation with food and eating, and the experience of feeling perpetually cold. Notably, when the participants in the Keys et al. study were allowed to eat freely, some of them engaged in binge eating when they were given access to food. Some even gained weight above their initial weight prior to the study, although most found that with time and access to food, their weight and eating patterns returned to normal.

This study is important for both patients and clinicians because it highlights the critical role of biological factors and nutritional status in triggering and maintaining binge eating. Specifically, inadequate nutritional consumption may elicit binge eating, perhaps an evolutionary remnant of ensuring overconsumption of energy following periods of famine or food deprivation. As a result, if patients remain malnourished through dietary restriction and/or purging, bulimic symptoms are likely to be perpetuated. For this reason, instituting planned meals and snacks that ensure appropriate energy intake and nutritional consumption are essential in providing a foundation for recovery from bulimic symptoms.

In addition to the Keys et al. study, which illustrates the importance of the biological factors of food deprivation in precipitating binge eating, research on dietary restraint (e.g., Herman & Polivy, 1975; Ruderman, Belzer, & Halperin, 1985) indicates that there are psychological factors as well as biological effects of food deprivation that can result in binge eating. Specifically, when individuals deprive themselves of "forbidden" foods (usually high in sugar or fat), they are more likely to overeat these foods when they are eventually exposed to them (e.g., in a party situation). This effect is especially pronounced when individuals classify "acceptable" and "unacceptable" foods in a rigid manner (e.g., "bad" foods). Based on this research as well as on several decades of cognitive-behavioral research indicating that targeting dietary restraint is critical to facilitate recovery from eating disorders (Fairburn, 2008), the clinician can emphasize the importance of not only consuming regular meals and snacks to prevent binge eating but also broadening the range of foods eaten. In particular, reconceptualizing rigid and dichotomous food classification and eating a broad range of food (including foods that might have been avoided and, as a result, consumed during binge-eating episodes) is especially helpful in preventing binge eating in response to the presence of avoided but desirable food. Eliminating these rigid classifications is especially relevant to ICAT-BN given that negative mood can enhance the effects of dietary restraint in eliciting overeating (Ruderman et al., 1985).

Another finding that can be shared with patients to provide a compelling rationale for meal planning is that several studies of CBT have found that individuals with eating disorders who have favorable outcomes often show significant change in the early phases of treatment that emphasize the consumption of planned meals and snacks (e.g., Wilson, Fairburn, Agras, Walsh, & Kraemer, 2002). Based on these findings, the introduction of meal planning early in treatment, including Phase II of ICAT-BN, appears to be particularly important for facilitating recovery from bulimic symptoms. Introducing meal planning early in treatment also provides the opportunity to provide exposure to strong emotions while simultaneously reducing avoidance behaviors. Because eating according to meal plans is distressing for many patients who fear weight gain, the process serves the additional purpose of eliciting strong emotions that can be the focus of treatment along with interrupting the bulimic cycle. In summary, eating regular planned meals and snacks is essential for recovery for both biological and psychological reasons and, based on previous treatment outcome studies in BN, appears to be an especially powerful intervention early in treatment.

Despite the importance of effective change in eating behavior early in the treatment of BN, many patients fear that the introduction of the CARE skill and meal planning will result in immediate and rapid weight gain. Thus, providing psychoeducational information (e.g., Handout 6.1) about the impact of meal planning and the ineffectiveness of purging is particularly important. Specifically, many decades of cognitive-behavioral treatment outcome research in which study participants have been encouraged to consume regular meals and snacks have indicated that the vast majority of participants did not gain weight (Fairburn, 2008). Explaining the ineffectiveness of purging in eliminating food consumed while overeating can help the patient understand why eating more frequently and, in most cases, having a greater amount of energy intake prevents binge eating without leading to weight gain. One of the most important studies to cite during Phase II when providing patients with a rationale for meal planning (e.g., Session 3, 4, or 5) is research that found that purging by vomiting does not eliminate all the food that is consumed during binge-eating episodes (Kaye, Weltzin, Hsu, McConaha, & Bolton, 1993). Specifically, these researchers studied individuals with BN in a feeding laboratory and analyzed the calorie density of participants' vomit when they had purged after binge eating. They found that only 50–70% of the food consumed was eliminated by vomiting, which suggests that individuals who self-induce vomiting retain 30–50% of the food eaten during the binge-eating episode. Similarly, laxatives and diuretics influence fluid levels but do not result in the elimination of actual energy intake. However, most individuals with eating disorders who purge experience a sense of both physical and psychological relief based on a false belief that they have counteracted the caloric intake of binge eating by purging. In addition, once the decision to purge has occurred, most individuals with BN report eating an increased amount with the anticipation of eliminating what has been eaten through purging (Fairburn, 2008). In discussing this information during Phase II sessions as well as by providing Handout 6.1, the clinician can help patients understand that by increasing energy intake through planned meals and snacks, they will reduce and sometimes even eliminate the urge to binge-eat; in addition, body weight is not likely to change (although there are exceptions), because purging does not eliminate food consumed and often leads to a larger ingestion of food while binge eating. Because the first part of Phase II involves establishing a compelling rationale before introducing the CARE skill, collaborative discussion to review self-monitoring and provide psychoeducation through handouts is particularly helpful in building the rationale. For most patients, two to three sessions in Phase II (e.g., Sessions 3–4 or 3–5) are often sufficient to help them understand the advantages of implementing meal planning. Although the psychoeducational information presented by the clinician, along with the handouts, provides a rationale for changing eating patterns, meal planning often elicits strong emotions and reluctance because patients often fear it will result in weight gain. Discussing the rationale in sessions is often quite helpful. Introducing these concepts when reviewing self-monitoring forms in the early Phase II sessions can be especially useful in personalizing the information for each patient. In discussing the rationale for changing eating patterns, include the following:

1. **Inadequate nutritional intake can serve as a biological trigger of binge eating.** Review Handout 6.1 to help patients understand that undereating contributes to their bulimic patterns, particularly the effects of semistarvation. Adequate intake prevents binge eating. Emphasize the negative effects of food restriction on undernourished patients, including mood disturbance and food preoccupation (Keys et al., 1950). To help illustrate this relationship, review examples of undereating followed by binge eating in patients' self-monitoring forms.

Example: "As I look through what you wrote, I notice that you tried not to eat much during the day and then ended up binge eating at night. It makes me wonder if one of the triggers for your binge eating is actually not eating enough during the day."

2. **Eating planned meals and snacks is one of the most powerful interventions to change binge-eating patterns (Fairburn, 2008).** In addition to providing Handout 6.1, the clinician can help educate patients about the several decades of research indicating that eating planned meals and snacks prevents binge-eating symptoms.

Example: "As we are discussing what happened yesterday, it's interesting to me that you ended up eating regular meals with your roommate throughout the day and didn't end up binge eating at night. In fact, this seems to be a pattern throughout the week: when you ate meals and snacks during the day, you were less likely to binge-eat at night. Your experience is supported by many years of research that has found that eating planned meals and snacks is very effective in reducing binge eating."

3. **Designating foods as "bad" and therefore to be avoided makes these foods more likely to become "binge" foods, which ultimately results in eating more (not less) of them.** Helping patients understand the risks of dietary restraint and beliefs about the need to avoid or restrict "bad" foods (usually designated as such due to perceived negative impact on weight/shape) can also help provide a foundation for changing eating patterns. In reviewing the self-monitoring logs, the clinician can note examples of this phenomenon when it occurs and educate the patient about the risks of assigning rigid food categories.

Example: "From what you wrote, it looks like you had decided to avoid eating all carbohydrates on Tuesday after you weighed yourself and were unhappy with the number. It's interesting that Tuesday night you ended up eating a lot of bread during your binge episode. Do you think there is a connection between trying to avoid carbohydrates and ending up eating them during binge episodes?"

4. **Purging by self-induced vomiting, laxatives, or diuretics often encourages binge eating but does not effectively eliminate food that is eaten.** Providing this information to patients helps them develop an understanding that their beliefs about purging to prevent weight gain from binge eating are erroneous.

Example: "I see that during the binge-eating episode you had last Saturday, you wrote that you 'decided to just keep eating and then get rid of it by throwing up.' Your thoughts about getting rid of what you've eaten by vomiting suggest that you believe purging is effective at ridding your body of whatever you eat. Would it surprise you to learn that your body actually retains a significant amount of what you eat even if you purge?"

INTRODUCING MEAL PLANNING USING THE CARE SKILL

After collaboratively discussing the rationale, the clinician introduces meal planning using the CARE skill and gives the patient Handout 6.5, "Meal Planning Using the CARE Skill." Given that patients often have strong emotional responses to the prospect of meal planning, reviewing this handout in session can be helpful because it provides an overview of both the concept and steps involved in meal planning. The overriding philosophy of meal planning in ICAT-BN is that moderation and variety lead to balanced eating and activity patterns, and that this balance is essential for general health and well-being. Meal planning also prevents impulsive eating and serves as a basis for self-care. In ICAT-BN, nutritional rehabilitation is viewed as an essential but often gradual process. Increasing the variety and overall amount of food consumed is emphasized along with frequency of meals and snacks as part of the CARE skill, which is outlined in Handout 6.2 and included in the skill cards.

The foundation of the CARE skill is to plan and eat meals and snacks that provide adequate nutrition. The implementation of the CARE skill will vary by patient. The clinician can use the early sessions of Phase II (e.g., Sessions 3–5) to establish in what ways and with what approach meal planning is most likely to be successful for a particular patient. For example, patients will vary in their ability to construct and implement a nutritionally sound meal plan. Some may struggle with knowledge about what types and amounts of foods to eat; others may "know" what to eat but may feel too fearful to increase the amount or variety of their food intake. The clinician can emphasize several main concepts of the CARE skill in collaborating with patients to develop meal-planning abilities:

1. Eating meals and snacks at regular intervals can reduce and prevent binge eating and purging as well as other types of compensatory behaviors (Fairburn, 2008).
2. Planning meals and snacks will eliminate "spur of the moment" decisions about eating that often lead to binge eating, purging, dietary restriction, and poor self-care.
3. Writing down meal plans (on paper or electronically) is extremely helpful.
4. Ideally, all food consumption after the introduction of the CARE skill in Phase II is planned.

Collaboration is critical to the implementation of the CARE skill. Many patients who have had previous experiences in eating disorder treatments describe having felt powerless and controlled by physicians, therapists, and dietitians (even well-meaning ones) in the context of meal planning. For this reason, the clinician should work with the patient to determine the appropriate level of comfort and risk taking. The potential conflict of guiding patients toward healthier food consumption while supporting their individuality and autonomy can raise potential challenges for the ICAT clinician. However, prescribing meal planning provides an ideal opportunity for the clinician to discuss these experiences as well as accompanying emotions. Being aware of this complexity and discussing these feelings directly can deepen therapeutic engagement, trust, and emotional self-awareness.

Ideally, the clinician can also strike a balance between being strongly empathic to the patients' fears about changing their eating patterns, while also emphasizing that the CARE skill is expected to elicit strong emotions. The CARE skill also serves to reduce avoidance of eating and build a foundation for eating patterns early in treatment. Although the CARE skill can be implemented gradually over the course of Phase II if necessary, the patient can also work toward changing eating patterns more rapidly. Encouraging rapid changes in the adoption of meal planning using the CARE skill has a number of advantages and is supported by empirical research (Wilson et al., 2002); however, some patients may need to change their eating behaviors more gradually.

Although the collaborative process and the patient's readiness will guide the introduction of the CARE skill, a typical session in which the CARE skill is introduced (e.g., Session 5 or 6) often proceeds as follows:

1. Review self-monitoring forms.
2. Review the rationale for establishing a regular eating pattern with planned meals and snacks: inadequate food intake triggers binge eating; many studies have found that eating planned meals and snacks reduces and prevents binge eating; changing eating patterns early in treatment often leads to better recovery (Handout 6.1 has typically been reviewed at a previous session).
3. Introduce the term CARE (as shown in Handout 6.2) and discuss Carefully Arrange Regular Eating concepts in detail (and provide Handouts 6.2–6.4).
4. Discuss specific strategies to start planning meals and snacks and make a collaborative decision about how to start.
5. Write down a plan for meals and snacks collaboratively for that day and the next several days using the version of the self-monitoring log called the "CARE Form" (see Handouts 6.3 and 6.4 and an example of a completed form in Figure 6.1).
6. Provide sample menus and discuss using them in a flexible manner if they are needed (see Handout 6.6).
7. "Check in" frequently about emotions that arise in the process of meal and activity planning and the anticipation of changing eating patterns.

MEAL-PLANNING DETAILS

As shown in Handout 6.4, the CARE skill involves detailed planning of both frequency and content of meals and snacks. In contrast to some CBT approaches (e.g., Fairburn, 2008), the patient is encouraged to establish a pattern of eating with three meals and two or three snacks, as well as ensuring that the content is varied and

CARE Form

Date _____

	PLAN	ACTUAL		
Time	Food/Drink	On plan (X) or actual	Type* (M, S, B, V, L, D, R, E)	Notes (feelings, skills used)
8:00 am	½ Bagel w/peanut butter (1 T) + butter (1 T), coffee (1 C), yogurt (1 C), 1 orange	X	M	At home, late for work
12:00 pm	Tuna and cheese sandwich, salad with dressing	X	M	At work, lunch meeting
3:00 pm	Banana milkshake, pretzels	Actual: nothing		Skipped snack—busy Worked late
6:00 pm	Pasta (1 cup) with chicken, Marinara sauce, and cheese; salad with dressing; small brownie	Actual: 8:00 pm Cereal (10 cups), Ice Cream (2 pts), Chips (family-size bag)	B	Got home late, upset, tried to eat snack but ended up bingeing
8:00 pm	Cereal (1 cup) with cranberries and nuts	Actual: 9:00 pm Milk (3 cups)	V	Feel full, sad, fat
Exercise (Type, duration):		None		

*Type: M = meal; S = snack; B = binge/overeating/eating more than planned/loss of control; V = vomiting; L = laxative; D = diuretic; R = restricting; E = exercise.

FIGURE 6.1. Example of a completed CARE form.

nutritious. However, the CARE skill also emphasizes flexibility without providing specific exchanges or amounts of macronutrient content. Given the ongoing debates about the optimally nutritious diet, the patient can be encouraged to experiment with guidance from the clinician. Reputable online information including *Choose-MyPlate.gov* can be recommended for individuals who struggle with generating meal plans (sample menus are also included in Handout 6.6); however, the patient can also be encouraged to eat avoided foods including desserts and educated about how these types of foods are, in fact, healthy to eat as part of a meal plan in order to prevent binge eating. Consider the following case example:

Example Dialogue

CLINICIAN: So now that we have reviewed the CARE skill and the rationale for establishing a meal plan, should we write down a plan for the remainder of today and tonight?

PATIENT: Well, I guess so. I mean, I am not sure exactly what to plan.

CLINICIAN: That's okay. Let's think about it together. So based on what I'm reading in your self-monitoring form for today, you ate breakfast. Have you had lunch?

PATIENT: No, not yet. I brought an apple for lunch.

CLINICIAN: That's a great start. Why don't you write that down on your CARE plan? What time do you want to eat it—as soon as you leave here?

PATIENT: Yes—maybe at 1:30?

CLINICIAN: That sounds good. As we've been discussing, eating an apple without anything else for lunch is likely to lead to more binge eating later. What else could you eat for lunch?

PATIENT: You mean like a sandwich or something?

CLINICIAN: Maybe. Do you like sandwiches?

PATIENT: No, not really. I do like soup, and I'll be driving by my favorite soup place on my way back to work.

CLINICIAN: Soup would be ideal. Is it a risky restaurant for you? A place where you have binged in the past?

PATIENT: No, I usually eat there with friends. But if I go there today, I would take it to go.

CLINICIAN: That sounds great. What size? What type?

PATIENT: I guess the large—chicken noodle is my favorite and they always have it. It comes with bread, but I don't usually eat it.

CLINICIAN: Wonderful. Do you want to try to eat the bread or is that too challenging?

PATIENT: I will try it. It's just a breadstick.

CLINICIAN: Great. So you'll eat back at your office at around 2:00?

PATIENT: Yes. I have some carrots there that I can eat too.

CLINICIAN: The plan sounds good. What do you want to plan to eat for an afternoon snack?

PATIENT: I don't usually eat one. Does it have to be like a snack food? Like chips or something?

CLINICIAN: No, not at all. Has anything worked well for you in the past when you were eating snacks?

PATIENT: Usually fruit and some almonds. I have almonds in my desk and a banana. I usually eat those for lunch, but I guess I could try them for a snack today.

CLINICIAN: That sounds like a good idea. Why don't you write those down? What time?

PATIENT: Probably after my meeting at 4:00.

CLINICIAN: Okay. What are your dinner plans?

PATIENT: Tonight is unusual. It's a friend's birthday, and we are going to her house for a barbeque.

CLINICIAN: Do you know what she is serving?

PATIENT: I think chicken and steak. I think I can eat those without any problems.

CLINICIAN: Wonderful. How much?

PATIENT: Maybe a piece of chicken and a small piece of steak. My friend likes salads, so I'm sure I can have some salads too.

CLINICIAN: How much salad?

PATIENT: Maybe I will plan to have one plate with the meat and salads. Usually she serves a pasta salad with cheese and green salad with dressing. Maybe a cup of both?

CLINICIAN: That sounds like a good plan. I imagine that they will serve dessert since it's a birthday party. What are your thoughts about that?

PATIENT: Too scary. I would end up wanting to throw up. I better skip dessert.

CLINICIAN: That sounds wise if it feels too risky. Finally, let's think about an evening snack. When will you have dinner?

PATIENT: Probably around 7:00. I'll get home around 10:00. Maybe a yogurt?

CLINICIAN: Fantastic. Let's see how that works for you. We can learn together as you experiment with meal planning. Eventually, we'll want to have you experiment with some riskier foods—things that you might typically eat during a binge, like dessert foods. For now, let's see how eating safer foods works for your CARE plan and what kinds of feelings you experience.

As illustrated by this example, the clinician collaborated with the patient to approximate a healthy meal plan. If the patient had struggled with ideas, the clinician could have used the *ChooseMyPlate.gov* website or Handout 6.6 to generate some menu ideas. Emphasizing experimentation and flexibility is essential as well as addressing feelings that arise in the session or occur in the context of meal planning. Although most patients with eating disorders find an emphasis on calorie counting to be unhelpful, the clinician can provide information about typical caloric needs (e.g., 2,000 calories/day) depending on energy expenditure, if necessary.

USING THE CARE SKILL
FROM THE MIDDLE TO END OF PHASE II

After the CARE skill and meal planning are introduced, the remainder of Phase II (Sessions 5–9) focuses on their successful implementation. Consistent with the early part of Phase II, sessions immediately following the introduction of the CARE skill typically include detailed review of the CARE forms, including planned eating and actual eating intake along with bulimic symptoms that may have occurred. Discussing situations in which the meal plan was not followed and whether or not this resulted in bulimic symptoms can be particularly effective. In general, the following themes should be considered toward the end of Phase II (e.g., Sessions 7–9):

1. **Situations associated with not following the meal plan and/or binge-eating symptoms.** Such situations include feelings and periods of nutritional deficits (e.g., inadequate intake). These situations can be discussed in the context of planning adaptive coping and introducing the ACT skill (see p. 103), especially for managing bulimic urges.

2. **Phase III concepts.** Relationship issues and self-evaluations that appear to precipitate bulimic symptoms can often be discussed in more detail in anticipation of Phase III, especially their role in triggering negative emotions and contributing to and maintaining bulimic patterns. This process sets the stage for Phase III and helps the patient continue to develop an understanding of the adaptive functions of binge-eating and purging symptoms for emotion regulation.

3. **Motivational issues.** When ambivalence is detected or motivational concerns arise, the clinician can use MI techniques from Phase I. For some patients, motivation remains a frequent focus of Phase II.

4. **Therapeutic rapport.** Rapport between the clinician and patient continues to be a preeminent goal.

5. **Emotional experiences.** Any explicit or implicit expression of emotions is important to emphasize and investigate during this phase.

After the introduction of the CARE skill, it is essential that the clinician provide explicit support and praise even very small accomplishments and behavior changes. Although some patients are able to construct and follow meal plans within several sessions, many struggle through much of Phase II and even Phase III. Consider this case example:

Example Dialogue

CLINICIAN: It is so helpful to read your notes about what you ate and how you were feeling during yesterday's dinner. Can you tell me more about what happened?

PATIENT: Yes, the day was going okay, and I was following my plan for breakfast and lunch and the afternoon snack. Then, I was at a party for dinner. I had planned to have a salad and a sandwich because that's what my friend said they were serving. But when I got to the party they had pizza instead. I tried to have a salad like I planned, but I kept smelling the pizza and thought I would probably be okay if I had one piece. But then I ended up having four and it just felt like too much, so I kept eating and ended up vomiting when I got home.

CLINICIAN: Yes, I see that you wrote about that on your form. And I also see that you wrote that you felt mad at your friend for changing the menu. That's a great use of the FEEL skill, especially in the midst of what happened. It also sounds like you did a great job of trying to follow the plan by having a salad when the menu did change. It seems like the pizza was really tough to have to face as a surprise.

PATIENT: It was, and I am upset about it because I made it the whole day before that following my plan and not binge eating or vomiting at all.

CLINICIAN: I know you struggled at dinner and the pizza really made it a challenge. I do want to point out what a great job you did writing out your plan, following it all day, and writing down exactly what was hard when you had to deal with the pizza, including your feelings. Also, it looks like you wrote down that in spite of the challenges of last night, you were able to get up this morning and eat your planned breakfast and lunch, and you haven't had any struggles today. That's a huge accomplishment as well.

MANAGING CHALLENGES WITH MEAL PLANNING

Several types of problems can arise in the context of meal planning in Phase II, illustrated in the examples in the following case scenarios.

Significant Dietary Restriction

At the beginning of Phase II, the patient described next was restricting his dietary intake significantly (1,000 calories per day or less) and eating a limited number of foods, based on fears that eating more in terms of amount, frequency, or variety would lead to weight gain. In this example, the clinician helps the patient devise a meal plan that is challenging but not overwhelming.

Example Dialogue

CLINICIAN: So, now we've reviewed the information on the handout and discussed the amount and variety of food that would be helpful to ensure that you are getting adequate nutrition, which in turn will help prevent your binge-eating and purging episodes from occurring. As we are talking here, I'm sensing that you are having some strong feelings. Can I check in with you about those?

PATIENT: Well, yes, honestly, I'm pretty freaked out about what you're saying— that I have to eat this much food? And even desserts?

CLINICIAN: When you say that you are feeling "freaked out," can you tell me more about what that feels like for you?

PATIENT: Well, I'm freaked out that if I eat all this I will definitely gain weight. And I haven't eaten dessert in years other than during binges. I can't even imagine doing it.

CLINICIAN: So you are feeling scared?

PATIENT: Yes. If I eat all of these meals and snacks—and variety, as you say—I will definitely gain weight. I hate being bulimic, but I don't want to gain weight.

CLINICIAN: I'm glad that you can label those feelings and that you are comfortable sharing them with me. We'll keep checking in about how you are feeling as we work together on this, but I am wondering if it might help if we approach making these changes in your eating patterns more gradually. For example, maybe it's too much to try to plan to eat dessert right now. What if we started writing some plans together that include foods you feel comfortable eating and that don't scare you quite as much? It would still be a challenge to eat more frequently, but the foods themselves will be less scary for you. It's important at this point that we work together to make sure that you are challenged in making changes, but that we don't push it if it feels like too much. How would that be?

PATIENT: Better, I think. Maybe I could try eating broccoli or something as a snack. That would make me nervous because I'm used to not eating all afternoon, but I think I could do it.

CLINICIAN: Great. Let's start writing down some plans, and we can include vegetables for your afternoon snacks. Also, I understand your concern about gaining weight, but since purging doesn't really eliminate the food that you consume, eating more regularly will actually prevent you from binge eating so you can incorporate more food into your meal plans and your weight is likely to remain stable.

Previous Familiarity with Meal Planning

This patient was in residential treatment several years ago when she was underweight but has not followed a meal plan since that time. Although she has maintained a body mass index (BMI) in a healthy weight range, she has continued to binge-eat and purge. The clinician helps this patient resume meal planning but with less precision than in her previous treatment in order to increase the emotional challenge and help the patient approach eating with less rigidity.

Example Dialogue

CLINICIAN: So now that we have reviewed the CARE skill and recommendations about meal planning, I want to check in to see how you are feeling and what you are thinking. As we were going through it together, I noticed that you were nodding in agreement at various points.

PATIENT: Yes, you know I worked with a meal plan back when I was underweight. I didn't like it at first, but it ended up really helping me. What you're describing here reminds me of what I did before.

CLINICIAN: So you're nodding because the meal plan makes sense to you and seems familiar.

PATIENT: Yes. Maybe it would help again. When I was in treatment before, I remember that I would measure out the food I ate for my meal plan and it helped me feel like I could control the details. It made me feel safe.

CLINICIAN: It sounds like meal planning helped you before and that you are comfortable trying it again. One thought I have is in response to your comment about safety. A goal of meal planning is to challenge you, to help you feel a little less safe, and to help you manage some of the feelings that may happen as you change your eating patterns. Would you be willing to experiment with following your plan without measuring your food?

PATIENT: I guess. It will be harder that way. I'll be scared that I am eating too much.

CLINICIAN: I understand that it will feel very different—both from how you are eating now and how you followed a meal plan in the past. Let's try it as an experiment and see how it goes. It will be especially important for you to write down your feelings and practice the FEEL skill as you try things out.

Frequent Purging Pattern

This patient eats unplanned meals and snacks throughout the day and evening on weekdays, often followed by purging. Binge eating occurs more frequently during the weekends. Although she consumes an adequate amount and variety of food, most eating results in purging. The clinician helps this patient understand the ineffectiveness of purging for weight control, the emotional function of the bulimic symptoms, and strategies for reducing the frequency of purging.

Example Dialogue

CLINICIAN: As we are reviewing the CARE skill and the meal-planning information, I'm wondering what you're thinking, and how you are feeling.

PATIENT: It makes sense, I guess. I mean, I think I already eat these foods. I eat a lot and I don't have any foods that I'm not "allowed" to eat the way it was when I was teenager. Now I don't avoid those foods—it's just that I'm used to purging after I eat them.

CLINICIAN: Yes, that's an excellent point and it's really helpful that you don't avoid certain types of foods. It seems like the bigger challenges will be doing the planning, and not purging after you eat.

PATIENT: Yes, both of those will be hard for me.

CLINICIAN: Hard in what way?

PATIENT: Well, I'm just used to purging. Then I don't have to worry about gaining weight. Although what we talked about last week—about that laboratory study that found that your body doesn't actually purge all the food you eat—that's made me think a lot about whether my purging makes sense. Every time I purge now I think about the fact that it's not really working, and that maybe I'm even eating more when I plan to purge, and I think I do. So purging doesn't seem like the great solution that it used to be for me.

CLINICIAN: Yes, I understand that. And from what you've written in your self-monitoring forms it sounds like when you don't purge, it ends up bringing up some feelings for you?

PATIENT: Yes, I get nervous about getting fat and I hate feeling full.

CLINICIAN: I'm glad you can identify that feeling of nervousness. It also helps us understand how the purging may be linked with your emotions. We'll continue to focus on those feelings as we work together on making some gradual changes. The most important parts of the CARE skill are the planning, and eating enough food and a variety of food without purging to ensure that you are getting adequate nutrition. How to go about doing that is usually based on personal preference. What do you think might work for you?

PATIENT: Maybe to try purging less?

CLINICIAN: That would be wonderful. Any thoughts about how you can make that happen?

PATIENT: Remind myself that it doesn't really work, and that purging actually makes me eat more.

CLINICIAN: Would you be willing to try writing down some plans for meals and snacks as well, just to see how it works?

PATIENT: Yes, I think so. As long as there is a choice built in—like saying I'll have a piece of fruit, and then I can decide if I want an apple or an orange.

CLINICIAN: Yes, that's a great idea. We'll make sure that there's flexibility built into each daily plan.

High Ambivalence

The following patient has been binge eating and purging for 10 years and came to treatment at the strong urging of her boyfriend. She expressed considerable ambivalence about giving up her bulimic symptoms during Phase I and has been inconsistently completing her self-monitoring forms during the early part of Phase II. The clinician works to increase the patient's motivation as well as suggesting a gradual approach to change.

Example Dialogue

CLINICIAN: So as we have been talking about the possibility of changing your eating patterns and why meal planning might be helpful, I'm trying to get a read on how you're feeling about that possibility.

PATIENT: Well, I don't know. I mean, it makes sense and everything, but it seems like a lot of work to write it all down ahead of time. And then how do I know if I'll even follow a plan if I have written it down?

CLINICIAN: So, I'm getting the sense that you might be feeling skeptical?

PATIENT: Yes, exactly. I mean, you know, it was my boyfriend's idea to come to therapy anyway. It's better than I thought it would be to come to these sessions, but I still don't think it's such a big deal if I'm only throwing up a few times a week.

CLINICIAN: If I understand what you are saying, in some ways your skepticism is about more than just the meal planning—in some ways you are questioning coming to treatment at all.

PATIENT: Well, sort of, I guess, although I do like meeting with you. And as much as writing stuff down is annoying, I have learned from that too.

CLINICIAN: What have you learned?

PATIENT: I thought I just purged out of habit, but when I look at what I've written down it seems like it happens when I'm upset. Like it's the way I deal with things.

CLINICIAN: Yes, that's well put. How has it helped to understand that pattern?

PATIENT: Well, I guess maybe there are other ways that I could cope, you know? Like why do I have to purge? Maybe there's a better way.

CLINICIAN: Yes, I understand what you mean. You see where you are now, and there's a part of you that really wants to be in a different place—for example, dealing with being upset in ways other than purging.

PATIENT: Yes, exactly.

CLINICIAN: And I guess that takes us back to meal planning, which is a strategy that we know can help with binge eating and purging. I hear that you have mixed feelings about meal planning in particular and about treatment in general, but you also don't like the fact that you purge when you are upset and want to find a different way of coping.

PATIENT: Yes.

CLINICIAN: One thought I have would be to experiment with meal planning in a more gradual way to see how it affects your eating, and especially your purging. We'll be able to see from your self-monitoring sheets if meal planning helps you purge less when you are upset. I wonder if it might work to try it between now and the next session. Should we jot down a few ideas about what you might eat for meals and snacks the rest of today, and into tomorrow?

PATIENT: Okay. I am willing to try it for a few days.

Frequent Self-Weighing

This next patient began to weigh herself following every meal and snack after meal planning was introduced. This weighing appeared to be based on a fear of weight gain.

Example Dialogue

CLINICIAN: It looks like you did such a wonderful job writing and following your CARE plan since the previous session. It also looks like you didn't have any bulimic episodes. That's great! What are the numbers in the column?

PATIENT: I weigh myself after each meal and snack.

CLINICIAN: Tell me about that.

PATIENT: Well, I know you said that the purging doesn't get everything out of my stomach, but I am just not used to eating so much, so often. I am really scared that I am going to gain so much weight.

CLINICIAN: Can you describe feeling scared? Is that happening right now?

PATIENT: Yes. Looking at my plan and how much I ate, I am just certain that the number will be up on the scale.

CLINICIAN: What does it feel like to be scared right now?

PATIENT: Like I am sort of shaky, my heart is racing. Like I have to do something, and weighing myself is the only thing that would help.

CLINICIAN: What is it like for you to sit with these feelings right now—to feel scared?

PATIENT: Really uncomfortable. When I get like that at home after I eat, I get on the scale.

CLINICIAN: So you found that weighing yourself was reassuring?

PATIENT: I guess—I mean, I felt 10 pounds larger after each meal, so it's a surprise to me that I'm not.

CLINICIAN: It does sound reassuring. And I also hear how awful it is for you to feel scared. But does weighing yourself sometimes make you feel worse?

PATIENT: Yes—and I get completely obsessed with it. I mean, I should know after a week that I feel bigger than the number. I don't know. Maybe the weighing doesn't reassure me because every little shift gets me completely upset.

CLINICIAN: Weighing is a tricky thing. Some people find that weighing themselves is helpful. It gives them data and helps make sure that they aren't avoiding their weight, which can make them even more anxious about it. However, weighing yourself after every time you eat sounds like it's making you feel worse. I wonder about cutting back on the frequency?

PATIENT: Yeah, that would probably help. Maybe I'll just weigh myself at the gym when I am there for class instead.

CLINICIAN: I find as we are talking that I am also wondering about using the FEEL skill after you eat. Maybe we can learn more about what it's like for you to feel scared.

PATIENT: Okay. I can try that too.

INTRODUCING THE ACT SKILL: ADAPTIVE COPING

Soon after the introduction of the CARE skill, the clinician can introduce the concept of adaptive coping using the ACT (Adaptive Coping Technique) skill as a way of managing bulimic urges.

As part of Phase II, patients learn about the problematic nature of behaviors that promote avoidance of emotion (e.g., food restriction, purging, binge eating). The CARE skill is thus not only a nutritional intervention but also an opportunity to face negative emotions without avoidance or escape. Providing patients with strategies to manage urges can further reduce avoidance behavior by facilitating effective coping skills.

The ACT (see Handout 6.7) skill directs the patient to several concrete and practical behavioral actions. It is important that these actions be simple, direct, and tailored to each patient. They are organized into three general categories: (1) self-soothing, (2) self-distracting, and (3) direct efforts to solve the problems that interfere with healthy eating behavior and elicit urges for BN behavior. One of the most important concepts in using the ACT skill in managing urges is to help the patient maintain a momentary focus. Patients can practice using these skills in the context of strong bulimic urges as well as during moments when they are struggling with following their CARE plan.

To introduce the ACT skill, the clinician can provide Handout 6.7 and discuss specific strategies that may be helpful. Discussing the ACT skill in the context of self-monitoring can be especially useful in providing the patient with concrete examples of how and when to implement this skill. Consider the following case example:

Example Dialogue

CLINICIAN: So tell me about what happened after work on Tuesday.

PATIENT: Well, I was about to leave work and I ran into my boss in the hall near the door. She said she had read the report that I had turned in and that it needed some work. We set up a meeting for the next day and it turned out okay, but I was really upset when I left work. I got in my car and I just couldn't calm down, and I started thinking about a binge. I knew what I wanted and I couldn't get it out of my head. I ended up driving to a fast-food restaurant and bingeing and purging. I could see what was happening. It's just like you and I have talked about. I end up bingeing and purging when I feel anxious—like I am going to get fired—and it helps in the moment because I don't have to think about what might happen. So I knew what was going on, but I still ended up at the restaurant.

CLINICIAN: It's such a great example, and I am really impressed by how beautifully you were able to track your feelings. I wonder if we should take a look at the ACT skill and see what might have been helpful for you. Do you remember the categories—self-soothe, self-distract, or solve the problem?

PATIENT: Yes, I was just looking over that list this morning. I wish I had thought of it at the time. But when I really think about how I was feeling after work and as I was driving to the restaurant, I was just so anxious that I don't think I could have solved the problem in the moment. I guess distraction might have worked.

CLINICIAN: What would have worked to help then? Another way to think about it is: What can you do to distract yourself when you are anxious in the future?

PATIENT: Honestly, talking to my friends is what helps me the most. I guess I need to just start calling people when I am anxious.

CLINICIAN: It might be helpful to even have a list of numbers programmed into your phone of friends who are especially soothing when you are upset. Would texting be even better?

PATIENT: No, talking on the phone or in person would be the best idea.

CLINICIAN: Talking to your friends sounds like a great distraction. Could you think of another way to calm yourself down—the soothing part? Let's think about how you could use the ACT skill for that.

INTRODUCING THE GOAL SKILL: GOAL SETTING IN TREATMENT

Phase II also includes goal-setting skills. Although some patients find this skill useful in the earlier part of Phase II, it is often optimal to discuss the GOAL skill (see Handout 6.8) after the CARE and ACT skills are developed (i.e., Sessions 5–8).

In introducing goal setting, the clinician can explain the rationale and steps as well as providing Handout 6.8. Specifically, the clinician discusses the value in setting treatment-related goals (e.g., practicing the FEEL skill for 10 minutes each day, writing a CARE plan each evening for the following day) to establish focus, structure, and momentum in attaining specific goals. The clinician also presents the importance of setting tangible and clearly defined goals as well as the importance of acknowledging goals when they are met. Typically, the clinician can collaborate with the patient in goal setting immediately after introducing this skill. The GOAL skill encourages patients to set realistic and helpful short-term goals throughout the various phases of ICAT-BN. Given the high self-standards that are so common among individuals with bulimic symptoms, the clinician's perspective is often helpful to ensure that goals are realistic. Goal setting is a collaborative process between the clinician and patient and can be reviewed and discussed at each session. The GOAL skill serves several functions in the context of ICAT-BN. First, because goal setting is an important aspect of emotion regulation (Thompson, 1994), the GOAL skill facilitates the establishment of short-term goals that provide motivation and fulfillment if reached. Second, it provides a forum to discuss self-standards, especially in Phase III. Finally, the GOAL skill provides momentum and reward as short-term goals are set in treatment as well as opportunities to understand potential obstacles.

In explaining the GOAL skill, the clinician can emphasize four primary components. First, the goal should be valued by the patient. Sometimes patients select goals that they believe others (e.g., significant other, family member, clinician) value. Collaborating to identify goals that are really important to the patient is essential. Second, the identified goal should be specific and measurable (e.g., "I will use the CARE skill to do meal planning every day this week before I go to bed"). Third, although long-term goals can be helpful (e.g., "My goal is to stop purging"), the GOAL skill in ICAT-BN typically emphasizes short-term goals that can be implemented and monitored on a daily or weekly basis. Finally, the clinician can focus on the importance of acknowledging the accomplishment of met goals or on learning from goals that are not met (e.g., using the CARE skill to meal plan after dinner rather than before bed if fatigue made completing the goal too difficult) in order to modify and identify more realistic goals.

Example Dialogue

CLINICIAN: Can we check in about your goal from last week?

PATIENT: Yes, my goal was to use my ACT skill plan every day, especially to stay distracted when I have urges to binge and purge at night after I get home.

CLINICIAN: How did it go?

PATIENT: It worked! I planned something distracting each night, and for several nights I went out with friends instead of coming home. I want to try the same thing for this weekend.

CLINICIAN: That sounds great. What an accomplishment!

DECIDING WHEN TO PROGRESS TO PHASE III

By the end of Phase II, patients are typically engaged with treatment and are using skills (i.e., FEEL, CARE, ACT, and GOAL) on a regular basis. Consistent meal planning is particularly important before progressing to Phase III. Some patients have experienced a dramatic reduction in bulimic symptoms by the end of Phase II; others may be highly symptomatic in spite of regular meal planning, treatment engagement, and skill use. Nonetheless, progression to Phase III is appropriate even for individuals with frequent bulimic symptoms. Moving on to Phase III can be delayed for patients who struggle with treatment engagement, as demonstrated by inconsistent session attendance, noncompletion of homework, and expressed ambivalence about treatment and change. For these individuals, resuming the MI techniques described in Phase I can help increase engagement prior to progressing to Phase III.

SUMMARY

The primary emphasis of Phase II is to introduce meal planning using the CARE skill for nutritional rehabilitation, symptom interruption, and emotional exposure. Typically, early sessions in Phase II focus on reviewing self-monitoring forms, identifying links between emotions and bulimic symptoms, understanding the function of bulimic behaviors, and developing a rationale for meal planning. Introducing meal planning using the CARE skill is a collaborative process in which the clinician remains attuned to emotions that often arise in the context of changing eating patterns. Phase II also provides an emphasis on the FEEL skill within and outside of sessions. Because the CARE skill is implemented in part to reduce avoidance behaviors, Phase II includes a focus on adaptive coping (ACT skill) and goal setting (GOAL skill) to help with motivation and self-regulation. In-session discussions and review of self-monitoring forms often function to set the stage for Phase III concepts and interventions.

Chapter 7

Modifying Responses to Situational and Emotional Cues (Phase III)

In Phase III, the focus of ICAT-BN shifts as the clinician and patient collaboratively identify the types of situations that precede problems in regulating one's emotions and subsequently lead to BN behaviors. This focus builds on the Phase I and II treatment components: enhancing motivation, helping the patient to identify emotions, planning meals and snacks, developing adaptive coping techniques, and learning goal setting. Clinicians need to encourage patients to continue to follow their CARE plan and to use the GOAL and ACT skills as they begin to address clinical targets in Phase III and learn new skills. As the patient becomes adept at identifying the links between situations, emotions, and their BN behaviors, he or she is encouraged to experiment with more adaptive choices to cope with distressing emotions "in the moment."

In this phase of ICAT-BN, clinicians focus primarily on the patient's interpersonal transactions, self-evaluative style, self-regulatory behaviors, food-related binge-eating cues, or a combination of these processes. The clinician and patient collaborate to understand how one or more of these four processes are linked to increases in negative emotions and subsequent BN behaviors. The relative importance of each of these areas for the development and maintenance of BN will vary in each patient, and therefore the primary therapeutic targets in Phase III will vary accordingly. The clinical targets in this phase are determined through the clinical formulation conducted at the beginning of Phase III and reviewed in the next section.

CLINICAL FORMULATION

Based on everything known about the patient at the beginning of Phase III, the clinician and patient collaborate to identify the cues for the patient's emotion dysregulation and bulimic behaviors. As can be seen in Figure 7.1, the clinician and patient can consider four distinct clinical targets and a fifth possibility that can involve more than one of these targets. Much of this information is summarized for the patient in Handout 7.1, "Choosing a Focus for Your Treatment."

Clinical Focus 1: Interpersonal Problems

The first clinical target involves *interpersonal problems*. This therapeutic target is chosen when interpersonal transactions are prominent as a cue for emotion dysregulation and bulimic behavior. Goals tend to involve modifying aspects of relationships that promote negative affect and BN behavior.

Case Example 1

Jenna is a 26-year-old marketing specialist with a 5-year history of bulimic symptoms. In the course of Phase II, she was able to eat planned meals and snacks and increased the variety of her food intake. However, she continued to experience bulimic episodes each time her boyfriend of 3 years went back to his apartment after they spent time together. Jenna described their dates as "intense" with ongoing disagreements about whether or not to get married. Her self-monitoring forms indicated that she would feel sadness and anger when her boyfriend would state that he was "not sure if and when" he wanted to get married, and that these feelings

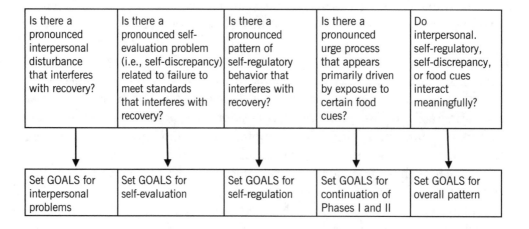

FIGURE 7.1. Developing a formulation and focus for Phase III.

typically precipitated her binge-eating and vomiting episodes. Jenna and her clinician agreed to focus on interpersonal problems as a clinical focus of Phase III and relied heavily on interventions related to the SAID skill and working on change in her relationship to her boyfriend.

Clinical Focus 2: Self-Evaluation

A second clinical target involves *self-evaluation*, most notably when there is a marked discrepancy between an individual's perceptions of her or his current self and desired or ideal personal standards. Such a focus on self-discrepancy may be seen in individuals with high levels of perfectionism and extreme goal setting that can figure prominently in bulimic behavior whether goals are related to appearance or other aspects of self-evaluation. Interventions based on self-evaluation tend to emphasize pursuing appropriate goals that are genuinely desired by the patient. Assisting the patient to effectively manage the disappointment of failing to reach a goal is also emphasized.

Case Example 2

Olivia is a 32-year-old lawyer with a 10-year history of bulimic symptoms. Although she has received numerous awards for her professional success including "Attorney of the Year" at her law firm, Olivia believes that she has not "lived up to" her standards for herself. For example, she had intended to publish a book and be appointed as a judge by the time she was 30. She also held extremely high standards about her weight and shape, for example that she "must always wear a size 4." In Phase II, Olivia was able to eat planned meals and snacks more regularly, including lunch, which she had typically not eaten because she was "too busy." This change in her eating pattern reduced the frequency of her bulimic episodes from daily to 2 days a week. Her self-monitoring forms indicated that these episodes typically occurred on the weekends when she was alone in the office. In the midst of working, Olivia would wander the halls and see other lawyers' certificates of achievement, which would elicit a sense that she had failed in her own self-standards. Highly distressed, she would binge-eat on candy from the vending machine. Olivia and her clinician agreed that self-evaluation would be their clinical focus in Phase III, and they worked on understanding her current standards and on using the elements of the REAL skill to work toward more adaptive standards.

Clinical Focus 3: Self-Regulation

A third clinical focus involves excesses and deficits in *self-regulation*, particularly involving high levels of self-criticism and self-control and low levels of self-protection and self-acceptance. Clinicians can choose this target if a patient displays bulimic episodes that appear to be elicited by periods of harsh, critical, and controlling self-directed behavior. Goals emphasize increased levels of self-protection and self-acceptance.

Case Example 3

James is a 20-year-old college student who has competed in elite track and field events since he was in sixth grade. James was recruited to his university's track team and was viewed as the "most promising" freshman. In order to ensure that he could live up to these expectations, James followed a strict diet and exercise regimen prior to starting college and had a very successful athletic season. During the summer between his freshman and sophomore years, James attempted to follow the same strict regimen of diet and exercise that he had pursued the summer before. However, he noticed that his athletic performance was not improving and, in addition, he experienced his first binge-eating episode at a fast-food restaurant near his summer job. Horrified by what he had eaten and its potential impact on his body composition and athletic performance, James self-induced vomiting and, although disgusted by his behavior, felt immediate relief in being able to "start over." James continued to attempt to follow his strict eating regimen and was extremely self-critical when he ate any food that contained gluten or refined sugar. His self-monitoring forms in Phase II indicated that his binge-eating episodes typically occurred when he was extremely self-critical and subsequently upset about his perceived failures in following his strict diet as well as not "advancing" as an athlete. In collaborative discussions of Phase III clinical targets, James and his clinician agreed to focus on self-regulation. Much of the treatment focused on his self-criticism and its function, with a deeper appreciation of learning self-acceptance and self-protection, skills.

Clinical Focus 4: Food- and Eating-Related Cues

The fourth target involves targeting *food- and eating-related cues* for individuals for whom these cues seem most prominent in triggering bulimic episodes. In essence, focusing on this category involves continuing Phase I and II work with an explicit emphasis on managing urges for bulimic behavior and developing more adaptive alternatives to responding to such urges. This option is chosen if it is determined that interpersonal problems, self-evaluation problems, and self-regulatory deficits, although possibly present, seem secondary to the potency of food-related cues in eliciting bulimic behavior. Established goals typically focus on having the patient monitor emotional responding and urges for binge eating when approaching eating situations that cue bulimic behavior and create a plan for adaptive coping. If the clinician and patient collaboratively agree that progress has been made regarding food cues and urges for bulimic behavior, additional momentary risk factors (e.g., interpersonal problems, self-evaluation) can be pursued in Phase III, but the emphasis should remain on food- and eating-related cues throughout the remainder of the treatment.

Case Example 4

Sarah is a 42-year-old administrative assistant with a 20-year history of bulimic symptoms. She is married and has two adolescent children. Her husband of 10 years works in a restaurant and brings home leftovers after his evening shift several nights a week. After her husband goes to bed, Sarah experiences overwhelming urges to eat these leftovers. She reports feeling "obsessed" with eating them once she sees and smells the food upon her husband's arrival. After he goes to bed, she binge-eats and vomits late into the evening. Sarah describes her marriage and work as fulfilling, and her self-monitoring forms in Phase II suggested that her negative emotions typically occur the morning after binge-eating episodes but rarely precipitate these eating events. Sarah was successful in implementing her CARE plan but continued to struggle with binge-eating episodes triggered by seeing and smelling the restaurant leftovers into Phase III. She and her clinician agreed to set goals related to food- and eating-related cues in Phase III, particularly using the CARE and ACT skills, as well as promoting emotion awareness through the FEEL skill.

Clinical Focus 5: Multiple Clinical Targets

The fifth possibility for clinicians to consider is that *more than one of these clinical targets* is important in precipitating bulimic episodes, and the clinician and patient agree that the combination of these risks can be meaningfully and effectively addressed in treatment. One particular combination we have noted is self-evaluation and self-regulation. In this combination, an individual with exceedingly high self-standards reacts to the experience of self-discrepancy with high levels of self-criticism and/or self-control. Typically, clinicians find it useful to assist such patients in not only modifying their standards, but also in considering alternative means of relating to the self. It is also possible, however, for other combinations to occur. Some patients may have difficult interpersonal relationships that significantly influence their self-evaluation. For example, if a patient has interpersonal difficulty with a given individual (e.g., parent, spouse, boss) and these difficulties seem to involve a perception of failing to meet the other person's expectations (i.e., a discrepancy between the self and another person's standards), it may be reasonable for the clinician to focus both on relationship and self-evaluation problems. Another possibility is the combination of extreme difficulties with food cues and self-evaluation. For example, some patients may have exceedingly high expectations regarding their ability to modify their meal planning, which leaves them vulnerable to food-related cues. Clinicians may find it useful in such a situation to continue to focus on the CARE plan, with a clearer emphasis on the individual's failure to meet standards regarding his or her ability to relate to food cues more adaptively.

Regardless of which target is chosen, it is important that the clinician and the patient come to a flexible agreement about the goals for treatment in Phase III and how they will proceed. Clinicians should emphasize that in a short-term treatment like ICAT-BN, such a focus is critical, and a collaborative agreement to maintain that focus both in and outside of therapy sessions is instrumental. Of course, if the initial formulation appears to be misguided, modifications can and should be made. As shown in the following example, selecting priorities for Phase III is a collaborative process guided by momentary data on emotional precipitants that have been identified in Phase II and the early sessions of Phase III.

Example Dialogue

CLINICIAN: So as we discussed last week, we will be shifting our focus in the next phase of our work together. You will continue to work on the CARE plan as well as trying to manage urges, but we will also focus on those things that seem to trigger your negative emotions and that lead to binge eating for you.

PATIENT: Yes, and I read through that handout you gave me about choosing the focus.

CLINICIAN: What do you think?

PATIENT: Well, I used to binge and vomit every day. I remember we talked at the beginning of treatment about how the first priority was to make sure I was eating enough because otherwise it could lead to binges. Eating meals and snacks has definitely helped, and now I am only having episodes on the weekends when I have to see my ex-husband. I know that I should be moving on from the divorce by now, but every time he picks up the kids on Saturday afternoon, I just get upset all over again.

CLINICIAN: I am noticing that you seem upset now as you are talking about it. Can you describe what you are feeling?

PATIENT: I just think about how he is with his new girlfriend, and how he seems happy now that he has left me, and I feel so furious and (*hesitates, tearing up*) sad too. Like he has someone, he still gets to see the kids, and I am going to be home by myself forever on Saturday nights. It feels like my heart is breaking and I am sick to my stomach. To be honest, if there were a cake in front of me right now, I would eat the whole thing.

CLINICIAN: I am really impressed by how you are describing your feelings, and sitting with them now here with me, in spite of how painful they are. I am also impressed by your awareness of how these feelings about your ex-husband are so strongly connected with urges to binge—even right here in the session. Based on what you are noticing and the fact that we have seen that your binges usually happen on Saturdays after your husband leaves with the kids, it sounds like focusing on your feelings about it and your relationship with him—and with other people too—would be really helpful for this next phase.

PATIENT: Yes, I agree. I think if I am wanting to binge on a cake right now sitting here in therapy, we are on to something with the relationship focus and how it triggers me! (*Laughs.*)

LINKING SITUATIONS AND EMOTIONAL STATES TO BULIMIC BEHAVIOR

Once the patient and clinician have identified a general area on which to focus in Phase III, they begin to look for opportunities to clarify how those particular types of situations influence emotional states and bulimic behavior. For example, if the formulation for a given patient focuses on interpersonal problems, the clinician and patient carefully review specific episodes of bulimic actions (e.g., binge, purge) for evidence of interpersonal problems that trigger emotion dysregulation and serve as a cue for the bulimic behavior. It is important for clinicians to recognize that such an assessment will look for proximal and momentary situational and emotional cues for bulimic episodes. In ICAT-BN, this complex of situations-emotions-actions is referred to as a SEA unit. Clinicians can help patients identify the SEA units that characterize BN episodes by using the SEA Change Diary. Once these SEA units are identified, the clinician and patient can collaboratively decide on how the patient might attempt to change the way he or she responds to those situational and emotional cues. Change can be made in a number of ways, for example, by modifying the amount of exposure to antecedent situations or by learning how to tolerate negative emotional states. Examination of the SEA units is central to determining the function of the BN behaviors and developing clinical targets. Understanding the cues that are most prominently involved in bulimic action not only informs the clinician about possible strategies for change, but also helps the patient to understand that his or her bulimic behavior is not random and is in fact a complex and patterned sequence of emotional and behavioral responses to high-risk situations.

The SEA Change Diary

The assessment of SEA units is conducted using the SEA Change Diary (Handouts 7.2 and 7.3). Patients are asked to record any instance of bulimic actions (e.g., binge, purge, restricted eating) during the recording period, which is typically the interval between treatment sessions. Clinicians and patients work collaboratively to identify the specific situations that preceded the bulimic behaviors (actions) reported by the patient and also search for the emotional state that preceded the episode. Because patients are continuing to record eating behavior on their CARE plan forms, they are not asked to provide a significant amount of dietary intake information in the SEA Change Diary. It is important that they provide specific episodes of bulimic action and, if they can, note situational and emotional cues that preceded the action. However, often the clinician will work with the patient in session to identify the situational and emotional antecedents to the bulimic episode that the patient is reporting. An example of a SEA Change Diary with hypothetical entries in all of the columns of the diary is shown in Figure 7.2. See Part III, Handouts 7.3 and 7.4, for a blank and sample completed SEA Change Diary for your patient to use.

SEA Change Diary

Situation	Emotion	Action
Had a fight on the phone with my sister after she canceled our plans	Sad Lonely Hurt Frustrated Abandoned	Bingeing instead of sticking with planned snack
What I needed in the situation/the function of the binge: I wanted a break from my life.		

Situation	Emotion	Action
Didn't get enough sleep last night, stayed up to watch TV	Bored Tired Guilty for almost falling asleep	Ate more than planned on during staff meeting then vomited after the meeting
What I needed in the situation/the function of the binge: Give myself something to do, keep me engaged in the meeting		

FIGURE 7.2. Example of a completed SEA Change Diary.

Patients begin to recognize key SEA sequences when their clinician repeatedly helps to identify the patterning of certain situations and emotions in cueing BN behavior. The example of Lindsay, a 21-year-old college student, demonstrates one such sequence.

Lindsay reported an instance in which she spent time with women in her sorority (situation), which led to feeling anxious and sad (emotion). In this instance, she left the social gathering and retreated to her dorm room, where she binge-ate and vomited (action).

Continuing with the SEA Change Diary review over several sessions, the clinician helped Lindsay to see this pattern across several additional episodes of bulimic behavior, and both agreed that her difficulties stemmed from unrealistic expectations about popularity and her appearance. The link between these self-standards and her emotions was explored in a manner that facilitated a heightened awareness of the depth of her feelings of sadness and anxiety but also helped her to see that continuing to pursue such unrealistic standards was counterproductive. Ultimately, Lindsay began setting goals to modify standards for herself, particularly regarding physical appearance. As she began Phase III of her treatment, she and her clinician began to focus on the nature of her standards for her appearance, the origin of these standards, and her expectancies regarding outcomes if she were to reach those standards. What evolved was an effort to change the way she evaluated her appearance by attempting to develop different appearance standards based on a broader perception of her sense of self. This modification led to an interesting shift in her friendship circle in which she was spending time with the women in her sorority who were less focused on appearance, which also helped her feel less isolated. Over time, this shift in friends and changes in her standards led Lindsay to be more accepting of herself.

Often the ICAT-BN clinician will already have ideas about a patient's key SEA units from the food logs the patient completed in Phase II. Over the course of several sessions, asking the patient to "walk back" from a BN episode through the preceding minutes and hours will reveal these central SEA sequences. The act of exploring these sequences helps one to "step outside" of one's life and notice the recurring patterns of situations that trigger bulimic behavior. Consider the following case example, in which Carla and her clinician begin to understand that when Carla goes home to her parents' house she is particularly prone to bulimic episodes. The clinician looks for the situational and emotional cues for this particular instance of bulimic action.

Example Dialogue

CLINICIAN: So you went home to your mom's house, and it sounds like you had a lot of trouble with your behavior. Let's start there.

PATIENT: Well, it was like it always is. I go home thinking it will be a clean slate and trying to start over and it seems like the minute I get in the door, she is criticizing me and trying to run my life.

CLINICIAN: Criticizing? Can you give me some examples?

PATIENT: Well, like when I got out of the car, she said, "You got a haircut. I liked it so much longer."

CLINICIAN: So, kind of picking on your appearance?

PATIENT: Yeah, all of the time. Every time I come home. She is always on me about my weight. When I was skinny, she would yell at me for being too thin. Now, she makes these snide comments about me eating too much at the table. On Saturday night, she literally didn't give me a dessert because she apparently thought I was too fat.

CLINICIAN: Yeah, it sounds like she's really focused on you and what you are doing. Take the example at the table and think about it for a minute. Tell me what that was like for you. What you were feeling as you were sitting in the chair. Try and focus on the sensations in your body and thoughts running through your mind.

PATIENT: Well, I could feel my neck turning red and I could feel a lump start to form in my throat. I know everyone was looking at me, and the only thought I could think was, I want to get out of here. I hate this place.

CLINICIAN: So you felt yourself getting kind of worked up, you felt like people were noticing, and you wanted to run.

PATIENT: Yes.

CLINICIAN: Like in the FEEL skill, let's see if we can find a good name or names for what you were feeling.

PATIENT: Well, I just felt so small and kind of embarrassed.

CLINICIAN: Was it embarrassed, like you had done something silly, or was it more like ashamed, like you felt bad about yourself?

PATIENT: I suppose I felt mostly just ashamed.

CLINICIAN: Anything else?

PATIENT: No, I don't think so.

CLINICIAN: I don't want to be too suggestive here, but did you resent your mother treating you this way?

PATIENT: You know I don't do anger well. That's not something I am very aware of, if it's happening at all.

CLINICIAN: Yeah, I've come to know that about you. Let's come back to that, but tell me, did you say anything when you were so ashamed?

PATIENT: Not really. My dad made a comment to my mom to give me some dessert and I just told him it was okay.

CLINICIAN: All right, so I am getting the feel of it, and I know that you had a binge-eating episode later that night. Help me understand what happened.

PATIENT: Well, it was probably an hour and a half later. I stayed at the table and just sat there.

CLINICIAN: Just sat there, or was something happening inside?

PATIENT: Well, at first I wanted to cry, but later I started drinking some wine at the table and I got angrier and angrier.

CLINICIAN: Tell me about the wine. Were you trying to settle yourself down?

PATIENT: No, I think I was trying to piss my mother off.

CLINICIAN: Did it work?

PATIENT: Yeah, by the end of the meal she wasn't talking to me. That was just fine.

CLINICIAN: So you think you were trying to get away from her?

PATIENT: Maybe. I didn't want to be there.

CLINICIAN: So then what happened?

PATIENT: Well, I went out and watched a little TV, but I was just sort of out of it, a little drunk. And then my parents went to bed. Then I started bingeing. It was just like I didn't care.

CLINICIAN: What do you think you were doing with the binge?

PATIENT: I think by then, I didn't care.

Once these sequences have been identified, the clinician and patient work collaboratively to develop a treatment plan for Phase III that flexibly addresses the clinical target.

WHEN SITUATIONAL CUES ELICIT "AUTOMATIC" BULIMIC BEHAVIOR

Typically, ICAT-BN attempts to identify and modify the relationship between triggering situations (e.g., interactions with people, events, times of day, sights, smells), emotional states, and bulimic behavior. However, sometimes patients will describe particular situations that reliably trigger bulimic behavior, but they cannot describe emotional states that connect the situation and the behavior. This pattern may be particularly apparent when foods or eating-related stimuli trigger a bulimic episode. For example, some individuals may identify a particular situation, like a food smell, a time (e.g., weekend), or visual cues (e.g., fast-food restaurant), that elicits strong urges for binge eating and any emotional component is either difficult to identify or clearly secondary to the situation. While ICAT-BN emphasizes the importance of carefully attempting to identify emotional correlates for such eating- and food-related cues, it is possible that certain potent environmental cues may trigger bulimic activity in what might be best construed as a habitual response. The premise that eating disorder behavior may become habitual, particularly after large numbers of symptomatic episodes occur in a predictable manner over long periods of time, is something many clinicians report. Recently, Walsh (2013) has advanced the idea that although the onset of anorexia nervosa (AN) may be heavily influenced by reinforcement and reward processes, including reducing negative emotions, the disorder may become significantly habitual over time and the reward functions appear less associated with the behavior than the cues that trigger the behavior. ICAT-BN acknowledges that this type of "habitual pattern" may also occur in BN and that BN episodes may represent part of a habit sequence that is largely triggered by environmental cues. Existing theories of habit behavior suggest that once a behavior becomes truly habitual, it is largely under the control of environmental cues and that the behavior represents a seemingly automatic, stereotyped sequence of behavioral routines that require minimal cognitive processing and are also difficult to inhibit (Verplanken & Orbel, 2003, Wood & Neal, 2007; Graybiel, 2008). In such cases, the SEA Change analysis in ICAT-BN may reveal situations that reliably elicit bulimic actions, but the emotional correlates of the sequence seem less significant to the patient. Later in this chapter, we describe specific procedures for dealing with what appear to be more entrenched habitual forms of bulimic action that are significantly influenced by powerful environment cues.

ICAT-BN INTERVENTIONS IN PHASE III

In Phase III of ICAT-BN, a number of interventions are utilized and new skills are introduced. A primary focus is assisting the patient in modifying situations that result in negative emotional states and increased risk of bulimic behavior. Figure 7.3 provides an outline of interventions for the primary types of interpersonal and

Interpersonal Problems	• Social Problem Solving • Promote Assertive Behavior
Self-Evaluation Deficits	• Promote Adaptive Personal Standards • Promote Realistic Appraisals of the Self
Self-Regulation Disturbances	• Reduce Self-Criticism and Self-Control • Increase Self-Protection and Self-Acceptance

FIGURE 7.3. Phase III ICAT-BN interventions.

intrapersonal situations thought to increase emotion dysregulation and lists the fundamental interventions for each type of situation.

Interventions and Techniques for Addressing Interpersonal Problems

As described in Chapter 2, individuals with BN often have significant problems in key relationships, both historically and currently. Early characterizations of individuals with eating disorders highlighted the interrelationship of relational factors, self-concept, emotion regulation, and eating disorder symptoms (Bruch, 1973). Furthermore, the observation that Interpersonal Therapy (IPT) has a significant clinical effect on BN (Fairburn et al., 1995), even without an emphasis on body shape, weight, or food, highlights the idea that interpersonal factors are intimately tied to BN. Additionally, the fact that empirical research has supported the fundamental tenets of the IPT model of binge eating suggests that interpersonal factors are important in BN (Ansell, Grilo, & White, 2012). Our experience has been that some patients will understand clearly that interpersonal relationships pose risks for BN behavior (and may benefit from reviewing Handout 7.5, "Beginning to Address My Relationship with Myself and Others" and Handout 7.6, "Possible Things to Change: My Relationships to Other People" in order to gain a clearer understanding of these problem areas). When attempting to modify interpersonal situations that trigger emotional dysregulation, there are two primary behavioral interventions: social problem solving and promoting assertive behavior. These two behavioral skills are considered elements in the SAID skill (described on page 122), which is designed to focus the patient and clinician on interpersonal problems and solutions to those problems. Each of these strategies will be reviewed below.

Social Problem Solving

The goal of social problem solving is to help patients generate new strategies to address and modify interpersonal problems. The following dialogue continues with Carla's episode at her parents' house (described previously) as the clinician uses the SEA Change Diary to facilitate social problem solving.

Example Dialogue

CLINICIAN: All right, we started to see this pattern, particularly with your mom, where you see her as critical and controlling and like you can never really do it right. It seems like you have become this little girl who alternates between apologizing and rebelling, but the whole time you seem to be feeling terrible, ashamed, and angry and eventually you just give up and sort of escape.

PATIENT: Yeah, I think that sort of sums it up.

CLINICIAN: Well, I am not sure what you will think of this, but I am wondering if you are interested in making any changes in the way you do things at home, and especially with your mother. Ever think about it?

PATIENT: Most of what I think about is just not ever going back, but I don't think I could do that.

CLINICIAN: Why not?

PATIENT: In some strange way I love them and I keep thinking that someday I will figure out how to make it right.

CLINICIAN: So in spite of it all, you still want to find a way to connect to them.

PATIENT: Yeah, I guess.

CLINICIAN: Well, let's talk about that. If you keep this pattern up, do you think you will ever get to that place where you can connect?

PATIENT: You mean with my mom criticizing and me feeling like crap? Not likely!

CLINICIAN: So let's talk about a different way. I'll try and get us rolling. One possibility would be to really just lay your cards on the table to both of your parents and tell them exactly how you feel when you are with them and when they treat you in particular ways. Tell them how it makes you feel and tell them how you would like it to be. This wouldn't be easy and it would probably be quite emotional.

PATIENT: Oh, I fantasize about it all of the time, but usually it's just telling them that they are wrong or they're bad and that never seems to be helpful.

CLINICIAN: Yeah, probably not. I am talking about something that's a little more open and genuine, but it would probably be really difficult and there's no telling what they'd do.

PATIENT: Yeah, I sometimes wonder if they will disown me.

CLINICIAN: Sometimes doing something like that is very helpful and people get closer, sometimes it doesn't do much good, and other times it can cause some difficulties.

PATIENT: Boy that sounds like a lot of fun. Got any other tricks in your bag?

CLINICIAN: Yeah, I got another one. You could pretty much disengage and separate. You can figure out how much of that you would want to do. Maybe cordial contacts at holidays, but not much else. Sort of designed to just protect you, and you take a stance that going there is not good for you and you have to protect yourself.

PATIENT: I think a lot about it.

CLINICIAN: Yeah, sometimes it's not a bad option. Not easy, but necessary in some situations.

PATIENT: I don't know.

CLINICIAN: Well, another possibility would be to just keep doing what you are doing or maybe step it up a little bit and get into some real knockdown drag-out fights. I don't know how it would work, but it could be pretty exciting! [Subtle humor?]

PATIENT: Probably not a good idea. I am not a good fighter.

CLINICIAN: Well, I am not big on helping people to fight either, so maybe we should think about some other options. Let's keep trying. What is coming to you?

This example illustrates how the clinician tries to engage Carla in social problem solving around the situation involving her parents. The summary of steps involved in this example of social problem solving is presented in Table 7.1. These steps are

TABLE 7.1. Steps for Social Problem Solving (for Carla)

1. **Identify the problem.** For Carla, this involves her interactions with her parents, particularly in their home.

2. **Define the problem.** Using SEA Change language, the problem seems to be that when Carla encounters critical and evaluative comments from her parents (*situation*) she feels ashamed, but also very angry (*emotion*). Her bulimic behavior seems to be a way to distance herself from her relationship to her parents, but also to let them know how upset she is (*function and action*). Defining the problem is likely to take place over more than one treatment session and should be carefully detailed by the clinician with numerous examples of the problem and the occurrence of the bulimic actions.

3. **Organize information.** Consider various strategies. As can be seen in the example, the clinician ultimately reaches a point where he asks Carla if she would like to consider doing things differently. Then he identifies several options (e.g., staying the same, aggressively fighting, disengaging or leaving, asserting), which are all discussed with Carla.

4. **Form a strategy.** Collaboratively try to find a solution to this dilemma. For example, Carla ultimately chose to basically stay the same, but to try to minimize her exposure to her parents and also accept the fact that their behavior is unlikely to change. She considered trying to assert her needs but decided the risks involved in this choice were not worth it.

5. **Implement the strategy and monitor progress.** For Carla, this choice will mean that she will need to deliberately go to her parents' house and try out the new strategy. She will need to monitor situational cues, emotional states, and urges for binge eating and alcohol consumption.

6. **Evaluate the results.** Carla and her clinician will need to talk about this clearly and openly. The problem they agreed to work on, based on the formulation, was her relationship to her family and its impact on her bulimic behavior. If the strategy chosen is ineffective, or causes unexpected problems, additional problem solving can be considered.

Note. Based on D'Zurilla and Goldfried (1971).

modified from the original D'Zurilla and Goldfried (1971) social problem-solving approach.

Promoting Assertive Behavior

Some patients with BN have great difficulty being assertive in interpersonal situations and may feel unable to interact with others in a manner that might lead to a more satisfying outcome. Clinicians can help these patients to learn assertiveness through in-session role plays. In these role plays, the patient engages in change-oriented conversations with the clinician, who often takes the role of the patient. Ultimately, some patients are encouraged to role-play as themselves after observing the clinician's demonstration of assertive behavior. In both cases, patients should be encouraged to be flexible in discussions with the other person while simultaneously adhering to the goals they have for that conversation. Patients should be reminded that interpersonal change takes time, that it is possible that their efforts may produce a positive outcome, even if not all goals are accomplished. It may also be important to understand that even the most skillful individuals may have some unsuccessful negotiations. Patients often find that being assertive can be emotionally satisfying regardless of whether the other person is influenced by the interaction.

Introducing the SAID Skill

Clinicians can assist patients to become more interpersonally effective by emphasizing the SAID skill, which stands for Sensitively Assert Ideas and Desires. As with all of the ICAT-BN skills, the SAID skill (Handout 7.7) represents a broad problem area that affects many BN patients—in this case in the realm of relationships with other people.

The following statements were developed by a patient struggling with assertiveness who wished to assert to another individual her desire to be less deferring:

> "I feel afraid of even saying these things because I feel as though I am not supposed to speak up. It seems like I am always trying to figure out what you want and then do it, even when it is not what I want at all. I want to be able to express myself to you more honestly even if you disagree with me. I'd like to know you think my ideas are valid. I have to say, it's hard for me to even tell you about this need of mine."

Other patients may not have trouble being assertive and instead tend to become angry and critical of others when feeling as though their needs are not met in a relationship. As shown in the following example, assertiveness and the SAID skill can be equally helpful for patients prone to aggression and verbal dominance as well as those who are prone to more submissive communication.

Example Dialogue

CLINICIAN: As you can see on this handout (*gives Handout 7.7 to the patient*), for the SAID skill it is important to be able to express your ideas and desires respectfully and effectively. What's your impression as you read through it?

PATIENT: Well, I don't have trouble speaking up for myself. Quite the opposite. I was raised to fight for my opinion. You should have seen our family dinners. It was all about debating politics and ideas. The loudest person, the one who could shout down everyone else, was considered the winner. In my most recent review at work, my supervisor told me that I had to learn to "tone down" the criticism that I give to my employees. That feedback surprised me—I binged after that meeting, actually, because I was so upset—because I thought that I was supposed to be a tough boss.

CLINICIAN: It sounds like based on your history, you learned to strongly express your ideas and desires. The tricky part, and it seems like it might be a challenge at work, is expressing yourself with sensitivity and respectfulness. Should we try a role play? Why don't you give me a recent example from your job?

PATIENT: Sure. I have to tell my assistant that she needs to go to advanced technology training because she doesn't seem to be mastering our new system. I don't know what her problem is, but I am tempted to go into the office and talk about her incompetence. Then I keep thinking about my review, so I haven't talked to her yet. But I really need her to take that class—not just for her but for our whole team so that we aren't slowed down by the new system anymore.

CLINICIAN: That's a great example. Okay, let's practice. I'll be you and you'll be her, all right? What's her name?

PATIENT: Her name is Jane.

CLINICIAN: Here I go, pretending to be you . . . Good morning, Jane. I was hoping to talk with you at some point today about some of our challenges with the new technology system. When would be a convenient time for us to sit down together?

PATIENT: (*Laughs.*) That is totally different from how I talk to her! Okay, sorry, this is actually really helpful to hear how you are saying it. Now I am pretending to be Jane. Um, I could meet now to talk.

CLINICIAN: Thank you. I would appreciate that. Could we meet in my office?

PATIENT: (*Pretending to be Jane*) Sure. Is there a problem?

CLINICIAN: Well, we are all facing a big adjustment with the new technology system. I wanted to ask if you would be willing to attend an advanced training seminar next week. I think it would be helpful to you in meeting the goals you have outlined for yourself in your recent job performance review as far as advancing your skills. It would also be extremely valuable to our entire team to have you develop expertise in the new system because you could help all of us with our own skills as well as working faster as a team.

PATIENT: Uh, okay. That sounds good. Can we be done with the role play? Wow, you sounded so nice as me. And as you were talking and I was pretending to be Jane, I didn't feel upset at all.

CLINICIAN: One strategy that I used in role-playing you was to imagine what this must be like for Jane, what she might feel comfortable hearing, and how taking the course might be helpful to her as well as for myself as her manager and for our team. I also used a tone of voice that was collaborative and not blaming. The point of the discussion, of using the SAID skill, is to express to Jane that you would like her to take a class, right? It's not to criticize her current performance. If that's your goal instead, you could do that in a separate meeting—again, respectfully, using the SAID skill.

PATIENT: Yeah, I get it. I will have to practice because talking like that is not natural for me, but I liked the way it sounded when you said it. If I talked more like that, work might be a lot easier for me if everyone isn't mad at me all the time and crying in the break room about what a tough boss I am. I think it's exactly what my manager meant when he told me to "tone it down." I thought that if I were too "nice," no one would do what I want, but I guess maybe a different way could work.

The Impact of Recurring Interpersonal Patterns on Phase III Work on Relationship Problems

While it is certainly possible for an individual to experience interpersonal problems with one key relationship, the more typical situation in ICAT-BN is that the patient will display a history of relationship problems. Often, the history of relationship difficulties is characterized by a recurring theme in which the patient displays a somewhat consistent pattern of interpersonal behavior. Some of the more typical interpersonal patterns emphasized in ICAT-BN include submission, withdrawal, unrealistic expectations of others, and blaming others. Relationship interventions in ICAT-BN address these enduring patterns. Patients may benefit from completing Handout 7.8, "The Development of Interpersonal Patterns," a questionnaire that helps identify the origins of these patterns. For example, an intervention for an individual whose primary pattern is submission may consist of identifying and expressing autonomous thoughts and feelings (perhaps using the SAID skill) as well as learning to adaptively tolerate interpersonal separations. Alternatively, individuals whose predominant pattern is to blame or criticize others may need to learn about the importance of empathy skills and try to develop friendly patterns of relationship, even when people do not fully comply with their desires. Handouts 7.5 and 7.6 may be useful to give to patients as they are clarifying the nature of their interpersonal difficulties. These handouts provide additional information about whether an individual's interpersonal problem is linked to a particular relationship or, alternatively, reflects a pattern of behavior across relationships. Patients can take them home, and clinicians should review the patient's thoughts about the content in the next session.

Ultimately, the goal is to attain what Benjamin (1996) considers an optimal style of interpersonal functioning characterized by moderate degrees of friendliness combined with moderate levels of interpersonal autonomy and the ability to rely on others when appropriate. Such a goal for relationships implies that individuals are clearly differentiated from others and able to make decisions or requests based on their own needs or desires, but also have the capacity to trust others and respect others' autonomy. Of course, it is important to emphasize that focusing on such relationship patterns should only be undertaken in ICAT-BN if the clinician believes the patterns are intimately linked to bulimic symptoms and that attempting to modify interpersonal behavior can impact bulimic episodes. Several of the more common patterns in BN (adapted from Benjamin, 1996) are described next.

SUBMIT PATTERN

A pattern frequently observed clinically, and described in empirical studies, is the submit pattern, characterized by a tendency to seek direction from others, passivity, and difficulties with autonomy and interpersonal separation. The goal of interventions addressing this pattern is to assist the patient to be more assertive and autonomous, while still being respectful and friendly. Interventions may also promote an increased tolerance for interpersonal separateness. Patients frequently resist such change because of fears that others will reject them if they do not behave submissively. Often, this interpersonal expectancy or appraisal is inaccurate, but there are clearly certain rigid or fragile relationships that may not tolerate such change, in which the patient's concerns are justified.

Techniques to facilitate change in a submit pattern include assertion training through role playing (as described in the preceding sample dialogue and in Handout 7.9). Specifically, patients with submissive patterns should be encouraged to identify genuine feeling states and thoughts, as well as their needs in relationships more generally or with a specific individual. This process may also involve sharing a desire or making a request of the other person, expressing negative feelings about the relation-ship, setting limits within the relationship, or expressing positive feelings toward the other person. In each session, clinicians will review interpersonal transactions with the patient in terms of whether or not different patterns of behavior were attempted. Typically this information is gathered using SEA Change techniques when interper-sonal situations are linked to BN behavior. If the patient does not display efforts to change and continues to engage in the same problematic SEA unit identified previ-ously, the clinician should attempt to identify obstacles to change, particularly in terms of fears or anxieties about negative outcomes if behavioral change should occur. When patients do engage in new patterns of behavior, the clinician should carefully review them with the patient in terms of their appraisal of the change and their emotional reaction to the new pattern of interpersonal behavior, as well as the interpersonal outcome. Obviously, if the outcome is positive for the patient the clinician can highlight the value of the change for the patient. However, in some situations behavioral change is not met with a positive outcome. In such cases, the clinician should clearly reinforce the patient's effort to make an adaptive interper-sonal change even if the other person involved did not provide a response that was rewarding. Many times patients need to be reminded that the absence of a favor-able outcome does not mean their behavior was inappropriate or unacceptable. It is possible that changes will be met with a negative response from others because the patient is no longer providing the expected pattern of behavior, which other people may have appreciated in spite of the fact that the pattern took a considerable toll on the patient.

WITHDRAWAL PATTERN

A second pattern frequently seen in individuals with eating disorders is the with-drawal or wall-off pattern in which the patient is significantly withdrawn from others, often with a certain amount of latent hostility and resentment. Such indi-viduals may be frightened about interpersonal intimacy or dependency but simul-taneously experience dysphoria about their high level of disengagement. Part of the problem may relate to expectations that all relationships are risky and should be avoided. Techniques for addressing this pattern include active encouragement of practice in social experiences and social skills training that highlights experiment-ing with approaching others and developing patterns of relating that include dis-closing appropriate personal information (see Handout 7.9). Some individuals who have significant withdrawal patterns will be quite reluctant to engage with others. Working with the patient to identify opportunities for engagement that are likely to be successful is a key. This may include individual relationships but can also include relationships with larger organizations and institutions (e.g., social clubs, religious groups). Preparing for such opportunities will also be important, with concerns and anxieties about approaching the relationship discussed thoroughly in the treatment with possible role-play experiences incorporated.

Occasionally, the withdrawal pattern involves a hostile and conflicted relationship with another person, and the patient will need to decide whether he or she wishes to discuss the conflict with the individual (utilizing the SAID skill) versus separating more fully from the relationship and attempting to "let go" of angry feelings. If the relationship has a fairly stable history and the other person appears able to tolerate a discussion of the feelings regarding the conflict, the former option may be preferable. However, if the other person appears to be unresponsive or hostile to a discussion of the difficulties, then helping the patient to resolve her or his feelings and minimize contact with the other person may be preferable.

PATTERN WITH UNREALISTIC EXPECTATIONS OF OTHERS

A third common pattern is in some ways similar to the submit pattern in terms of autonomy deficits, but there is a clear expectation that others will care for and tolerate individuals who demonstrate this pattern. The basic idea underlying such behavior is that others either "will" or "should" take care of them, which is unfortunately often met with ambivalence or resentment from others. Addressing the hope or the expectation that others will take care of the patient can be challenging clinically. The primary strategy will be to discuss clearly the particular relationships in which the pattern is occurring and the transactions that are typical of the relationship. If it is clear that the other person in the relationship (e.g., significant other) is frustrated or angry by the patient's expectations, working with the patient to gain some empathy and understanding regarding the other person's reaction may be useful. Also, considering with the patient the possibility that the other person may withdraw from the relationship because of the patient's demands and expectations provides important and realistic information. Collaborating with the patient on beginning to assume a greater level of responsibility for his or her behavior and promoting and rewarding evidence of such autonomous action by the patient are essential. The fundamental concept that should be encouraged in these situations is that the patient can expect to have close and supportive relationships with others, but that it is optimal if such attachments are coupled with a clear respect for the boundaries of other individuals and efforts to learn skills that promote the patient's autonomy (see Handout 7.9).

Occasionally, clinicians will identify a pattern in which the patient may hold unrealistic expectations for the clinician. For example, a patient may expect that the clinician will conduct treatment "on the patient" that will facilitate change or recovery without the patient's active involvement. Also, a patient may expect that clinicians will solve other extraneous problems in the patient's life, such as resolving interpersonal difficulties with significant others or employers. Regardless of the particular type of situation the patient hopes the clinician will resolve for them, the important point is to promote the collaborative focus of ICAT-BN and assume the patient will work with the clinician and responsibly make changes in his or her life. Clinicians should be careful to not gratify patients' wishes or expectations excessively, but at the same time understand that the patient's expectation needs to be addressed sensitively and empathically.

BLAME AND CRITICIZE PATTERN

A fourth pattern observed in some individuals with BN is the blame pattern. In this pattern, the patient is likely to use blame and criticism, perhaps to influence significant others. Unfortunately, such individuals do not recognize that such hostility often results in others withdrawing from them, which may not be the desired outcome (Benjamin 1996, 2003). These patients may benefit from exploring their actual wishes and desires in relationship with other key people, and the ineffectiveness of blaming others in achieving these goals. In essence, these patients need to gain a clearer understanding of the interpersonal sensitivities and needs of others and the negative effect of their hostile demands on the interpersonal availability of others (see Handout 7.9). Techniques commonly used will include empathic confrontation of the patient's blame pattern, including an exploration of possible underlying dependency, fear of aloneness, or chronic feelings of being misunderstood. In the end, the most essential point to introduce to the patient who uses blaming and criticizing patterns is that such patterns are most likely to result in the loss of relationships and support, which is often not the intent of the patient. If that is not the patient's ultimate goal, attempting to inhibit such actions and develop alternative skills for relating is essential. Unfortunately, this pattern may be difficult to modify, and addressing the pattern may increase the chance of the patient dropping out of treatment.

In summary, patients with problematic interpersonal patterns may benefit from referring to Handout 7.8, "The Development of Interpersonal Patterns," which is a questionnaire designed to help the patient gain a deeper understanding of the origin of his or her interpersonal patterns and the functions they may have served historically and currently. Handout 7.9, "Tips on Modifying Interpersonal Patterns," is a series of practical tips and suggestions for modifying interpersonal patterns. The handout is organized according to the particular patterns just discussed with specific recommendations for each pattern. Each of these may inform the therapeutic dialogue but also provide additional experiences outside of session that can help patients continue to work on modifying their patterns of behavior.

Finally, clinicians may find that the treatment of patients with significant interpersonal problems and patterns that are clearly linked to bulimic episodes may benefit from the inclusion of significant others in sessions. In the ICAT-BN randomized controlled trial, significant others were not included in the protocol. However, in clinical practice this may provide useful information about interpersonal issues in the patient's life and also the degree to which significant others can be seen as meaningful resources in the treatment. However, in ICAT-BN, the rationale for bringing in a significant other would be that interpersonal problems or patterns have been clearly linked to bulimic episodes and the clinician believes the inclusion of a significant other would help modify this momentary risk factor. Inclusion of significant others for generic psychoeducation regarding BN or simple support of the patient may be clinically appropriate, but are not technically included in ICAT-BN.

Interventions and Techniques for Addressing Self-Evaluation Deficits

In their original publication "Binge Eating as Escape from Self-Awareness," Heatherton and Baumeister (1991) discuss escape theory and link binge eating to a variety of other behaviors that share a common function of avoiding painful awareness of the self and associated negative emotional states. Fundamental to escape theory, however, is the notion that individuals escape from self-awareness when they compare the self against high standards or ideals they feel they have failed to meet. The authors state, "A first prediction is therefore that binge eaters will be characterized by unusually high standards, including goals, perceived expectations, and ideals" (p. 89). ICAT-BN similarly emphasizes the experience of failing to live up to standards and ideals as a significant factor in the onset and maintenance of BN behavior.

As described in Chapter 2, ICAT-BN emphasizes self-discrepancy theory (Higgins, 1987), a model of self-regulation and emotions that focuses on the relationship between one's perception of one's actual self and one's personal standards—against which the self is evaluated. Within this theory, two types of personal standards are emphasized. The first standard reflects an individual's perception of an ideal self, or the person he or she *wishes* to be. A second type is the ought standard, which reflects an individual's sense of responsibility and obligation, the type of person he or she *must* be. Discrepancies between the actual self and the ideal self have been found to be specifically associated with sadness and dejection, whereas discrepancies between the actual self and the ought self are typically associated with anxiety and worry. In the ICAT-BN model, bulimic patients are thought to display significant discrepancies between the actual self and both ideal and ought standards. In ICAT-BN, in order to facilitate simpler therapeutic communication with patients, the ideal and ought standards have been collapsed into one "desired" standard. Because discrepancies regarding physical appearance, shape, and/or weight are often important for individuals with BN, these types of discrepancies are emphasized in ICAT-BN, as well as more general self-discrepancies that do not involve appearance.

It is important to emphasize once again that self-discrepancy in the ICAT-BN model is particularly significant from a momentary perspective. That is, although certain patients may have traits characterized by high levels of self-discrepancy, ICAT-BN attempts to emphasize those moments in time in which self-discrepancy occurs, particularly as it triggers negative emotion. Depending on the clinical focus, the ICAT-BN clinician will be looking for self-discrepancy-oriented moments preceding negative emotions associated with bulimic behavior. The following example highlights self-discrepancy:

Example Dialogue

PATIENT: My body felt so ugly to me this week. Fat and disgusting.

CLINICIAN: That sounds important. Can you tell me when you were noticing it?

PATIENT: Well, yesterday, when I was at the beach with my boyfriend I noticed it. My boyfriend says he doesn't notice, but I know I look disgusting.

CLINICIAN: It makes me think about our discussion last week, of looking at the discrepancy, or the difference, between how you see yourself as you are, and how this is different from how you want yourself to be.

PATIENT: Yes, my ideal is to have a completely flat stomach. Anything less than that is fat and disgusting.

CLINICIAN: So in terms of your desired self, it's about having a flat stomach. That's what you really want?

PATIENT: Yes, exactly.

CLINICIAN: Well, let's talk about who you wish you could be. What's it like to think about your flat stomach?

PATIENT: I haven't had a flat stomach for years, maybe never. I don't know. I just want it to be flat.

CLINICIAN: Yeah, I see, but how does having this standard of a flat stomach affect you?

PATIENT: It makes me feel disgusting. It makes me feel like I have to restrict, and like I have to purge each time I eat.

CLINICIAN: So when you compare your stomach to the ideal you feel bad and your bulimic behaviors get worse.

PATIENT: Yes.

CLINICIAN: Yeah, when there is too big a gap between how you see yourself and how you want to see yourself, we find people feel worse. What about changing your standards? Ever thought about it?

PATIENT: I don't know. It feels like giving up.

CLINICIAN: Well, in a way you would be letting go of something. In doing that you may feel some disappointment or maybe confusion, but the idea would be to come up with a new goal for how you want to be. Maybe one that doesn't leave you feeling so frustrated.

PATIENT: What you say reminds me of people who buy lottery tickets.

CLINICIAN: In what way?

PATIENT: You know, they don't have enough money, but they spend too much on lottery tickets each week because they have this dream that they are going to win. But they never do.

CLINICIAN: That's a great example. And how does their ideal of winning the lottery affect them?

PATIENT: Well, they are upset each week when they don't win, and they spend money.

CLINICIAN: What would you recommend to them?

PATIENT: Change their goal about winning the lottery.

CLINICIAN: Could that flat stomach ideal be your version of winning the lottery? Could that ideal be changed too?

PATIENT: Maybe it could.

Clinicians should attend to these discrepancies and when they believe that a patient's momentary emotional experience is related to a perceived failure to live up to self-standards, these standards should be targeted directly.

Promoting Adaptive Personal Standards and Realistic Appraisals of the Self

ICAT-BN interventions and techniques to modify problematic self-evaluation are designed to promote personal standards that reflect an understanding that the goal is to pursue valued standards that are attainable without harming the self. Furthermore, ICAT-BN encourages an ability to tolerate disappointment when personal goals are not met. A series of strategies for addressing self-discrepancy are outlined in Table 7.2. The first step in self-discrepancy-oriented interventions is to identify the standard that is not being met (e.g., not thin enough). A second component is to examine the relationship between pursuit of the individual's personal standards and his or her emotional experience. For example, on a momentary basis, do negative emotional states precipitate and intensify the pursuit of the personal standard?

On the other hand, does pursuit of the standard result in worsening or an improvement in emotional experience? A third component in these interventions is to identify the patient's expectation regarding the attainment of the personal standard. In other words, what is the expected reward that an individual anticipates if the standard is achieved? As can be seen in Table 7.2, it may also be useful to ask questions about the history of the standard. Did the standard emerge during a time involving certain particular activities or relationships? Why might it have developed at that time? It may also be useful to ask patients to attempt to identify the potential costs of pursuit of such a standard. Do they recognize that the pursuit of such high-level standards may take a behavioral toll on the individual? Finally, when the patient and the clinician have a clear understanding of the momentary and historical antecedents and consequences of the standard, they may begin to discuss change and develop new, more adaptive standards. Often, relinquishing such standards is extremely difficult for patients because of fears that alternative and more adaptive standards would reflect "giving up" and may be associated with negative consequences (e.g., social rejection). Consequently, change of self-standards may often be a very gradual process in which the standards are examined and questioned.

TABLE 7.2. Steps for Addressing Self-Discrepancy

1. Clearly identify the standard that the patient is attempting to achieve.

2. What is the relationship of the personal standard and the individual's emotional experience (both historically and in terms of current momentary states)?
   - Does negative emotional experience precipitate increased pursuit of the standard?
   - Does pursuit of the standard reduce or intensify negative emotional experience?

3. What does the patient expect will occur if the standard is attained? What will be the reward?

4. What is the history of the standard?
   - When did this standard become so important?
   - Why did it gain importance when it did?
   - Do these standards influence the patient each day?

5. What is the potential cost to the patient for pursuing this personal standard?

6. Does the patient entertain the idea of beginning to change personal standards?

7. Based on the person's current experience and true motivations, what standards would he or she like to pursue?

Introducing the REAL Skill

The REAL skill is intended to address deficits in self-evaluation and facilitate change in self-discrepancy. Self-discrepancy involves unrealistic standards for the self. The REAL skill may also be useful in helping the patient identify devalued or disavowed aspects of the actual self that are thought to be unacceptable or inadequate. The goal of self-discrepancy reduction is to help the patient develop more reasonable evaluative personal standards and expectations for the self while simultaneously growing in acceptance of the actual self.

The essence of the REAL skill, depicted in Handout 7.10 and included in the patient's skill cards, is to carefully consider the impact that negative self-evaluations can have on the patient. Patients are encouraged to carry the skill cards to remind them of the core principles of the REAL skill. Handout 7.11, "Possible Things to Change: Expectations for Myself," and Handout 7.12, "What Do I Wish to Be?" provide both descriptive information about the notion of self-discrepancy and its impact on people and also a series of questions to clarify personal standards and values for the patient. In particular, these worksheets are meant to help patients understand more fully the significance of negative self-evaluation in a person's life and begin to develop more adaptive personal standards. Handout 7.13, "Checking My Personal Standards," provides a worksheet designed to encourage patients to carefully consider their specific standards and delineate them in writing. Completion of this exercise, along with the other worksheets, may provide useful insights for the patient that can be discussed more thoroughly in therapy sessions. Such worksheets should also be shared with the clinician to deepen the value of the therapeutic dialogue.

Interventions and Techniques for Addressing Self-Regulation Disturbances

In ICAT-BN, the focus on self-regulation bears certain similarities to evolving work in psychotherapy focusing on self-compassion. For example, Gilbert's theory of, and treatment for, depression and other forms of psychopathology highlights the role of self-criticism, self-directed hostility, and shame in emotion dysregulation and psychopathology (Gilbert, 2009, 2010). Recently, compassion-focused therapy has also been considered and used in the treatment of eating disorders, with some evidence of utility (Goss & Allan, 2014; Kelly & Carter, 2014). Although not evolving from the same theoretical background as these approaches, ICAT-BN does highlight the importance of hostile self-control and self-criticism as triggering and maintaining factors in BN and also targets increasing self-directed behaviors such as self-protection and self-acceptance, particularly as a person is attempting to recover from an eating disorder.

In ICAT-BN, as the clinician reviews SEA Change Diary data with the patient regarding situations that precede bulimic actions, he or she may begin to notice patterns of behavior directed toward the self. They will hear phrases such as "I hate myself," "I can't believe what a loser I am," or "I won't let that happen to me." These statements are clear examples of self-criticism or extreme self-control that are referred to in ICAT-BN as self-directed behavior. In ICAT-BN, such self-directed behavior is thought to be triggered by negative emotion, and patients engage in such behavior because they expect it will be helpful, but typically it worsens emotional states. The goal of ICAT-BN is to reduce such extreme self-criticism or self-control and promote the development of greater self-protection and self-acceptance.

Reducing Self-Criticism and Self-Control and Increasing Self-Protection and Self-Acceptance

A first step in modifying self-directed behavior is to conduct a careful functional analysis of the patient's self-directed behaviors. As with the interventions and techniques addressing self-discrepancy, the clinician attempts to identify the relationship between various self-directed behaviors and emotional states. Do episodes of critical or controlling self-directed behaviors follow or precede negative emotional experiences? For example, do patients experience a reduction in negative emotions after being self-controlling or self-critical? On the other hand, does their emotional state actually worsen after periods of self-criticism or self-control? A second step requires identifying the patient's expectancy regarding the potential value of such self-directed behaviors. For example, do patients anticipate that by being self-critical they will motivate themselves to achieve goals or personal standards that are extremely hard to attain? Simply put, what is the purpose of hostile and controlling self-directed behaviors? Third, the clinician may help the patient to assess whether the self-directed behaviors *actually* help the patient. Do they work? Are there unforeseen consequences? Do these self-directed behaviors potentially increase the risk of bulimic behavior? Finally, clinicians can collaboratively discuss the possibility of alternate ways of relating to the self, including self-protection and self-acceptance. Self-protection is clearly defined as making efforts to not put the self in a position of risk or harm, including high-risk bulimic behavior situations (e.g., skipping meals). Self-acceptance refers to an effort to tolerate and accept the self, in spite of perceived insufficiencies and inadequacies. Like many other changes pursued in ICAT-BN, such efforts may proceed very gradually and with considerable ambivalence or difficulty. However, the potential value of reducing hostile self-control behaviors and promoting a more protective and accepting relationship with the self can be an important component of recovery. The clinician may use the sequence of steps outlined in Table 7.3 to address self-regulation problems.

TABLE 7.3. Steps for Addressing Self-Regulation Problems

1. Identify what types of situations and emotions precipitate self-criticism and self-control.
   - Do negative emotional states trigger maladaptive self-directed behaviors?
   - Do self-criticism and self-control improve or worsen the emotional well-being of the individual?

2. What is the patient's expectancy regarding engaging in self-criticism and self-control?
   - Does the patient expect such self-directed behavior will enhance performance, appearance, or general well-being?

3. Does it work for the patient to engage in such self-criticism and self-control? What are the payoffs?

4. Do self-criticism and self-control have negative consequences?

5. Is the patient interested in trying to develop a less hostile and controlling relationship toward him- or herself?
   - Does the patient understand the nature of self-protection or self-acceptance?
   - Would the patient like to practice a lifestyle in which such self-directed behaviors occur?

Introducing the SPA Skill

The fundamental purpose of the SPA Skill (Handout 7.14) is to have patients pay careful attention to the nature of behaviors such as self-directed criticism, control, or neglect and to understand the purpose of the behaviors. Most patients with BN do not engage in high levels of self-acceptance or self-protection. The clinician and patient can collaborate to identify patterns of self-directed behavior associated with negative emotional states as well as to understand the function of these behaviors. The clinician may assess whether the patient understands the idea of self-protection and self-acceptance. For example, reliably following a meal plan may be construed as a self-protective behavior for a BN patient who is trying to recover, but such self-protection may be quite unfamiliar to many patients.

Additionally, clinicians may attempt to promote the practice of self-acceptance (e.g., tolerance of appearance) or self-protection (e.g., carefully following meal plans and not engaging in risky, neglectful behaviors that are known to precipitate binge eating). Given these long-standing patterns, such adaptive self-oriented behaviors may develop quite slowly over the course of treatment.

Example Dialogue

CLINICIAN: Okay, so let's see, you had a binge and purge episode on Saturday and one of the things that I notice is that you spent several hours before you began binge eating restricting and exercising, and it seems you were trying to eat as little as possible. Is that right?

PATIENT: Yeah, I think that's probably true. Maybe I overdid it a little bit.

CLINICIAN: Well, let's look at it. I am curious to know a couple of things about the exercise and not eating. How did you decide to do that? Had something occurred or was there a thought going through your head earlier in the day?

PATIENT: Well, I had gone home the day before and saw some of my old friends.

CLINICIAN: What was the visit like?

PATIENT: Well, it was sort of mixed. It was nice to see them, but I always leave feeling somehow inadequate. One of them is getting married. One of them had just been accepted into graduate school and the other one was preparing for a marathon and had lost a bunch of weight. I don't know, I just felt not so great.

CLINICIAN: Was it a comparison thing where you felt like you weren't accomplishing what they were doing?

PATIENT: Yeah, probably.

CLINICIAN: Tell me about that. What were you experiencing?

PATIENT: I just felt kind of empty, like a loser. [A longer discussion about the emotional reaction is limited here for readability.]

CLINICIAN: Well, let's think about that. Then you began exercising the next day. Do you think there is any connection?

PATIENT: Well, I am not sure. I do know that I just thought if I could lose a few pounds, I would be accomplishing something. I think I just wanted something to happen that was good for me.

CLINICIAN: So maybe part of the exercise and not eating yesterday was about trying to improve yourself and achieve a goal, at least from your perspective. So in a way, you were really trying to steer yourself in a direction that you hoped would be good, but it didn't quite work out that way. Does that sound right?

PATIENT: Yeah, I think so. It seems like it never does work out.

Often, the patient recognizes that his or her self-directed behavior is ineffective or counterproductive. Nonetheless, it is important to place the patient's self-regulatory behavior in a functional context and to appreciate that the patient's behavior is an effort to manage a problem. Usually this effort can be validated as an effort to improve the patient's life, but with a maladaptive strategy. It is important to point out that there are several handouts that can be given to the patient to supplement therapeutic sessions. Handout 7.14 provides a version of the SPA skill that can be used in conjunction with the skill cards. Handout 7.15, "Possible Things to Change: The Way I Treat Myself," provides an overview of the notion of self-directed behavior and different ways in which an individual can treat him- or herself. Handout 7.16, "Tips on Changing the Way You Treat Yourself," on the other hand, offers practical ideas about modifying patterns of self-directed behavior. Each of these handouts can be provided to the patient during appropriate therapy sessions and reviewed in ensuing sessions in a manner that facilitates therapeutic discussion.

Interventions and Techniques for Addressing Situationally Triggered BN Habitual Behaviors

Some patients' BN behavior seems largely triggered by situational cues that involve food-related stimuli. The simple smell or sight of certain high-risk binge foods may prompt extremely strong urges for binge–purge behavior. Also, cues associated with the food, such as the sight of a fast-food restaurant that prepares highly desired binge foods, may be sufficient to trigger binge–purge behavior. Often, such patients are conceptualized in a Phase III formulation that emphasizes the food cues and deemphasizes emotional triggers such as interpersonal, self-evaluative, or self-regulatory factors (see Figure 7.1). The example of Sarah, at the beginning of this chapter (Case Example 4), describes an individual who experiences such powerful situation-driven behaviors.

As noted in Figure 7.1, many of the techniques and interventions initiated in Phase I and Phase II of ICAT-BN may be continued in Phase III for such individuals without other interventions addressing other interpersonal or intrapersonal factors. That is, the primary emphasis is placed on managing the response to particular situational cues (ACT skill) and developing an alternative food- and eating-related behavioral repertoire (CARE skill). Thus, there may be a significant emphasis placed on improving awareness of triggering situational cues and developing alternative action plans in the face of such cues. Clinicians help the patient to gain a clearer understanding of the explicit situations that are likely to trigger bulimic behavior and develop more concrete, behavioral plans in the face of such cues. Also, ICAT-BN may promote interventions to minimize exposure to such high-risk cues (e.g., avoiding driving routes past fast-food restaurants). In ICAT-BN, emotional awareness training (i.e., FEEL skill) might continue to be significant for such patients, particularly as they try to change their responses to triggering situational cues. Patients may have distressing emotional experiences as they engage in new behavioral patterns in response to such cues and awareness, identification, and expression of these emotional states in treatment can be useful.

In general, the recommended intervention for individuals who appear to have environmentally cued, habitual binge–purge behaviors is to develop different habits and behaviors in response to high-risk cues. Concrete, explicit, and simple behavioral strategies to utilize when exposed to triggering cues comprise the fundamental treatment and resemble contemporary habit-reversal interventions (e.g., Watkins & Nolen-Hoeksema, 2014; Woods, Himle, & Conelea, 2006; Wood & Neal, 2007). These interventions will require careful delineation of the most potent environmental cues that seem to trigger binge eating or purging. Such cue awareness training may be conducted by completing a SEA Change Diary but remaining focused on only the situation and the action, without examination of emotional correlates. The goal would be to help the patient identify those situations that are particularly significant in terms of cuing urges and bulimic episodes. Once the situational cues are clearly identified, the clinician and patient together identify a concrete behavioral response to the cue that is not bulimic behavior. In ICAT-BN terminology, this is essentially implementation of the ACT skill, but it is important that it be simple and easy to perform in the face of motivationally significant cues.

Example Dialogue

CLINICIAN: It is really beginning to look like certain types of cues in the environment increase the chances of having a binge. Particularly, driving by a fast-food restaurant that sells French fries and also going to the cafeteria in your dormitory when they are serving pasta.

PATIENT: Yeah, it seems like I can be doing really well and then if I smell French fries or see pasta in just about any form, I have real trouble. It seems like it becomes automatic and I just can't stop it.

CLINICIAN: Yeah, it sure does. Let me tell you what we typically do when people have these kinds of automatic triggers for their bingeing. First, we really work on trying to be aware of cues. The basic idea is to prevent you from getting caught off guard. So, if the two cues we want to work on are French fries and pasta, we would need to really heighten your awareness of when you might encounter these situations. It might mean being aware of the restaurants that are the greatest risk in terms of exposure to French fries and being aware of your location in relation to them. It might also mean being very aware of when they might be serving pasta in the cafeteria and knowing the times that you are at greatest risk.

PATIENT: Yeah, I really don't seem to pay careful enough attention. I just sort of go about my business and before I know it, it is just happening.

CLINICIAN: Yeah, it is sort of hard to be aware of these things, but we think this can be learned. The second step is trying to come up with a real concrete alternative response if you do encounter situations where there are fries or pasta. Let's think about what we could do with that. If you are with a group of friends and you are going into the cafeteria or are making a decision to go to a restaurant and they pick one with French fries, what could you use as a plan to protect you? I think of it as sort of a frontline survival skill for when you get exposed to one of your cues. We find that knowing clearly what you will do differently when you see the trigger and then having it right at your fingertips is the best plan. Too much thinking in that kind of situation can be a problem.

PATIENT: So it sounds like you think I should come up with something that I could easily do if I am aware that I am in trouble and want to try and prevent a binge.

CLINICIAN: Exactly! Let's try and flesh that out, but remember, let's keep it simple and doable.

PHASE III TROUBLESHOOTING

Clinicians are likely to experience a number of common challenges as they work through Phase III with their patients. In this section we explore these challenges and offer some therapeutic strategies for meeting these difficult clinical moments.

The Patient Does Not Complete the SEA Change Diary Outside of Session

Patients often are willing to report bulimic actions but do not record them in real time.

1. Revisit the purpose of the SEA Change Diary. It is an opportunity to describe the patient's life as it is happening. Patients are unlikely to use this worksheet if they see it as a useless exercise and do not understand the rationale.

2. Model use of the SEA Change Diary in session. If the patient would like to discuss some event that occurred between sessions but did not complete a SEA Change Diary on that event, the clinician can pull out a blank worksheet and say, "While you are talking about this, I'd like to sketch out what I am hearing and then we can look at the diary and see if it is helpful in understanding what happened. How does that sound?"

3. The clinician can explore with the patient what gets in the way of using the SEA Change Diary and then with the patient engage in problem solving those barriers.

The Patient Is Willing to Try Changes but the Bulimic Behaviors Keep Occurring

Another common and often difficult problem in this phase is that while patients might be willing to attempt interpersonal, self-evaluative, or self-regulatory changes, they struggle to give up the reliable emotional relief they get from engaging in BN behaviors. Suggestions for helping patients with this struggle include:

1. Join with the patient in acknowledging that there are many good reasons why restricting, binge eating, and purging have worked in terms of changing aversive feelings. Validating the important function of these behaviors can help the patient feel accepted and may lead to increased willingness to try new ways of behaving again.
2. Explore the benefits and costs of the BN behaviors, either briefly or in more extended MI. This strategy is also another way of joining with the patient and can just take the form of a simple reminder of things that have been learned in previous sessions. For example, a clinician might say:

"You and I have talked about how a late-night binge can really help you avoid the feelings of panic you get when you are alone at night and feeling overwhelmed. You have also told me that soon after a binge, the panic gets replaced by self-loathing, which feels even more painful to you. Sometimes you have been able to self-soothe at night by putting on your favorite song and taking a bath. Are you willing to explore what got in the way this night with doing something like that?"

The Patient Fears Loss of Self-Control If Personal Standards Are Changed or Self-Acceptance Is Practiced

Another common problem encountered in Phase III is that the patient is very fearful that any move toward greater self-acceptance or developing more moderate standards will lead to lack of self-control. This concern is also understandable if patients have been using self-criticism and pursuit of high standards as an attempt to feel more in control of their lives for many years. One patient told her ICAT-BN clinician that if she became more self-accepting, she would end up like the obese mother in the movie *What's Eating Gilbert Grape?* who had not left her house in 7 years. The patient had a very strong visual image of herself becoming like this character. Clinicians may wish to try some of the following strategies to help patients with this fear of losing control in the face of making change.

1. Validate patients' fears and acknowledge that their personal standards and their ways of treating themselves have served an important function.
2. Explore the function of these thoughts and behaviors again as well as the emotions associated with them.
3. Ask patients to try in session, for a few brief moments, to entertain the change (greater self-acceptance or reducing self-discrepancy) and, using the FEEL skill, discuss what emotions are evoked.
4. Ask patients to set up an hour (or more) between sessions to act "as if," meaning they will treat themselves in a more self-accepting way or change their standards for that time period and see how that feels. Once the time period is over, they can go back to their old way of being.
5. Ask patients if they would prescribe their way of being for a loved one or dear friend. Generally patients will say they would not, and the reasons they would not can be explored.
6. Ask patients if there was a time in their life when they did not treat themselves with criticism or excessive control and whether that resulted in being "out of control" as feared.
7. Ask patients to visit the times they are actually "out of control" now despite their extreme personal standards or attempts at self-control through harsh thoughts about the self or maladaptive behaviors.
8. Walk through the suggestions in this chapter for introducing the REAL and SPA skills.

The Patient Fears Using the SAID Skill to Change Interpersonal Situations

Patients who have trouble with assertiveness are almost, by definition, fearful about trying the SAID skill. On the other hand, there are some patients who display anger in an attempt to control the behavior of others. They too can benefit from using the SAID skill, though they may fear that doing so will be ineffective or they will "lose" something in the process.

1. Validate patients' fears and acknowledge that trying out a new behavior is often difficult at first.
2. Explore patients' past experiences with any successful behavior change. Consider metaphors like sports or music. For example, what was it like when they first learned a sport? How did they learn to be adept at a sports activity or playing a musical instrument? Patients will likely relay that it took practice and shaping their behavior over time. Ask the patient if learning the SAID skill might be the same as learning other new skills.

3. Use the SAID skill during in-session role plays.

4. Ask patients to practice the SAID skill with a safe person in their life.

5. Ask patients to practice the SAID skill in easier situations first. Create a hierarchy of situations with patients, starting with situations where it is easy to be assertive and ending with those where it would be extremely difficult. Ask them to try some of the easy ones before the next session and complete a SEA Change Diary on the attempts.

6. Ask patients if there is someone in their life who they see as very skillful in self-assertiveness. Can they imagine themselves as that person when they try the SAID skill? Would the patient be willing to ask the skilled person to coach them in practicing the steps in the SAID skill?

SUMMARY

Phase III of ICAT-BN is focused on reducing affect dysregulation by modifying exposure or response to situational cues that precipitate emotional difficulties and bulimic behavior. Clinicians and patients collaboratively develop a formulation of the primary cues for bulimic episodes and target these cues throughout Phase III. Three areas of momentary cues are emphasized in ICAT-BN, including interpersonal experiences, experiences of maladaptive self-evaluation, and self-regulation. Additionally, some individuals with BN may be cued for bulimic behavior by powerful environmental cues, with responses that resemble habitual behaviors. The primary focus of Phase III is to reliably identify the cues that promote bulimic behavior and work to modify the impact of those cues on the patient's emotional experience and behavioral responding.

Chapter 8

Stabilizing Treatment Gains and Termination (Phase IV)

The primary goals of ICAT-BN Phase IV are to consolidate improvements made in treatment, provide strategies to prevent relapse, and end treatment collaboratively. Consistent with previous ICAT-BN phases, the clinician maintains a strong focus on emotions within the sessions as well as those emotions the patient describes as having occurred between sessions. Although Phase IV includes skill acquisition with the introduction of the WAIT skill (Watch All Impulses Today), much of this learning is facilitated through homework and review of the handouts rather than through didactics during the sessions. An emphasis is placed on a balanced, healthy lifestyle along with a keen awareness of the role that various life situations, emotional responding, and maladaptive actions have had in the patient's history of binge eating and purging, along with strategies to continue action patterns that support self-care.

CONTENT OF PHASE IV SESSIONS

Typically, the transition from Phase III to Phase IV begins with the final two to four sessions of treatment. At this time, the clinician can explicitly discuss with the patient that the final phase of ICAT-BN will provide an opportunity for reviewing, planning, and ending treatment collaboratively. In addition, the clinician can emphasize the importance of relapse prevention and continued treatment progress. The structure of these final sessions typically involves a gradual reduction in the time spent reviewing self-monitoring and SEA Change Diaries during the session. Some patients may choose to continue to complete these forms even after treatment is finished. Near the beginning of Phase IV, the clinician can explain that some people choose to stop and others choose to continue various types of self-monitoring. If the patient decides to discontinue self-monitoring, ideally this change can be implemented with at least two sessions left before termination in case this change leads to an increase in symptoms or distress. Other patients may decide to continue a modified self-monitoring system using their calendar, cell phone, or computer. Experimentation can be encouraged, with an emphasis on examining how reducing or eliminating self-monitoring impacts both behavior and emotions. Given how central self-monitoring and SEA Change Diaries are to the ICAT-BN content and focus, the formal cessation of these procedures can be associated with strong feelings, either negative (e.g., fear, anxiety) or positive (e.g., relief), which can be discussed during Phase IV sessions. For those who decide to stop (which, in our experience, is most typical), the clinician can suggest that restarting CARE plans, self-monitoring, and SEA Change Diaries is a helpful strategy in times of potential future struggles or lapses. As demonstrated in the example below, experimenting with changes in self-monitoring prior to the end of treatment can be useful in case the patient struggles with the transition.

Example Dialogue

CLINICIAN: So, we are wrapping up treatment in the next few weeks and we are now moving into the final phase of our treatment together. Did you have a chance to read the handouts I gave you last session?

PATIENT: Yes, I did.

CLINICIAN: One of the decisions we can discuss is whether you want to continue completing CARE plans, self-monitoring forms, and SEA Change Diaries on your own after our sessions have ended. As I am talking, I can see that you are having a response to what I am saying. Can you tell me what you are feeling right now?

PATIENT: (*Laughs slightly.*) Well, if you had told me 3 months ago that I could stop all this homework I would have been thrilled because it was so hard to do at the start. But now that I am used to it and my eating is so much better, I am kind of scared to give it up. I mean, I should be relieved that I can stop but instead, I am nervous.

CLINICIAN: Can you tell me more about feeling nervous?

PATIENT: I guess it's more a worry—like what if I start throwing up again because I'm not writing everything down? I don't really think it's likely because it's been so long since it's happened and I don't even really think about throwing up anymore, but what if I am doing so well because of all of this writing and focus? Still, I am kind of excited too—to see how I do. It's almost like leaving the nest—both my sessions with you and all of the forms. I kind of want to try it. It's funny, because as I am talking about stopping the forms I am actually feeling less nervous and happier, especially about not needing to hide them from my coworkers anymore. That will be a relief.

CLINICIAN: So, you are nervous but also excited about using this final phase of treatment to experiment without SEA Change Diaries, CARE plans, and self-monitoring. Perhaps we can try having you stop using them for this week as an experiment. If the first couple of days go smoothly, you can try for the whole week; if you notice trouble tomorrow or the next day, you can go back to the forms and try something more gradual—like keeping track on your personal calendar instead. How does that sound?

PATIENT: Good! I like the idea of trying it. It will feel weird but freeing to not worry about hiding them. I am excited to try it tomorrow. (*Smiles.*)

INTRODUCING THE WAIT SKILL

Early in Phase IV, the clinician can use Handout 8.1 to introduce the WAIT skill (Watch All Impulses Today). The WAIT skill helps maintain the "momentary" focus through the final phase of ICAT-BN and beyond termination. This skill emphasizes the importance of momentary self-awareness and builds from what has been learned through self-monitoring and the SEA Change Diaries from earlier phases. One of the other important features of the WAIT skill is that it is not limited to bulimic symptoms but can be used for other potentially problematic impulses (e.g., substance use) as well. As illustrated in the following case example, it often helps to discuss the WAIT skill in the context of specific examples.

Example Dialogue

CLINICIAN: In discussing the WAIT skill, it sounds like you are most concerned about evenings after work. Can we talk more about that? You think that evenings might be the time when you are most likely to have a lapse and end up binge eating and purging?

PATIENT: Yeah, that's when it used to happen and I still sometimes have urges. It's one of the reasons that I try to go out with friends after work to prevent it from happening. But if I am stressed out from work and I come in the door and go to the refrigerator, I am afraid that the next thing I know, I'll have food all over the kitchen. It's been quite a while since I've done it, but I'm afraid it might happen if work gets too busy.

CLINICIAN: That's a great example, and it's really helpful that you already know that evenings after work are a high-risk time. I think it's why the WAIT skill will be so useful. By keeping track of your impulses, you can be aware of them and come up with an effective strategy to either soothe yourself or distract yourself to prevent the bulimic symptoms from happening. Also, continuing to do the ACT skill in those moments is really helpful.

PATIENT: Sometimes the desire to binge and purge seems to come out of nowhere.

CLINICIAN: Yes, and that's why the WAIT skill emphasizes watching your impulses or urges in the moment. If you are aware of and tracking your urges, you won't be as likely to be caught off guard. Often, what feels like an urge coming out of nowhere might actually have been building more gradually. Using the WAIT skill can help you be aware of urges early on and make it easier to use the ACT skill to prevent a bulimic episode.

Patient: Yes, that's probably true. It used to be in the afternoon that I'd actually start thinking about or even planning a binge, many hours before I left work. I guess that would lead up to the strong urges to binge and purge after work.

CLINICIAN: Yes, exactly. With the WAIT skill, you can be aware when it's happening, and as you mentioned before, go to a friend's house after work if you are having urges.

PATIENT: Will I have to do this forever—like always being on guard?

CLINICIAN: It's most important to be especially self-aware right after treatment ends. Most people find that with continued success, self-awareness becomes easier and urges continue to decrease. But in some respects, continuing to use the WAIT skill on an ongoing basis will be useful—especially if things are stressful at work. The idea isn't to be anxious about it. It's about being watchful, self-aware, and maybe even curious about how are you feeling in the moment.

PATIENT: Yes, that makes sense, and a lot of stuff that seemed hard when I first started treatment—like planning meals—now seems automatic. Maybe watching myself in that curious way will become more automatic too.

RELAPSE PREVENTION

One of the primary aims of Phase IV is to establish relapse prevention strategies, given the high rate of relapse in BN (see Chapter 2; Mitchell et al., 1985b; Olmsted, Kaplan, & Rockert, 1994). Relapse prevention in Phase IV includes education about the process of relapse, healthy lifestyle planning, introduction of the WAIT skill, and consolidation and continuation of treatment progress. Within this context, the clinician can continue to emphasize the potential function of eating patterns in response to emotions as well as strategies to continue to engage in different action behaviors when triggering situations and accompanying emotions arise.

Educating the patient about the nature of relapse is an important initial step. By the end of treatment, many patients are quite confident about the progress they have made and may even be surprised to hear that they are at risk of becoming symptomatic in the future. Conversely, others believe that they "will always have an eating problem," even when they are no longer symptomatic. The clinician can explain that individuals who no longer experience bulimic behaviors may in fact be free of symptoms for a sustained period of time, or even permanently; however, they can expect to encounter potentially challenging situations that put them at high risk of relapse, especially in the first year following treatment. These struggles, while challenging, can be viewed as valuable educational experiences (Fairburn, 2008; Fairburn et al., 1993b). Because of the risk of relapse in BN, it is important for patients to identify their own risk factors and plan to maintain their success over time. The clinician can emphasize that the patient can continue to make progress after the end of treatment, as well as emphasizing the potential for lapses being used as learning experiences.

One of the most important concepts for patients to understand is the difference between a "lapse" and a "relapse" (Fairburn et al., 1993b). A "lapse" or slip is the occurrence of a minor symptom, while a "relapse" refers to a recurrence of frequent binge eating and purging. Because a lapse is a single event, it does not necessarily lead to relapse (Brownell, Marlatt, Lichtenstein, & Wilson, 1986). As outlined by Marlatt and Gordon (1985), the individual's response to a lapse can determine whether it escalates into a relapse. If an individual has very strict rules about maintaining abstinence from symptoms (i.e., is highly self-controlled), a lapse can precipitate what Marlatt and Gordon (1985) describe as the abstinence violation effect, in which the individual experiences guilt and self-blame about his or her perceived "failure." The abstinence violation effect consists of both the cognitive attribution of the cause of the lapse and the affective response to this interpretation (Grilo & Shiffman, 1994). The greater the intensity of the abstinence violation effect, the greater the likelihood that the lapse will escalate into a full-blown relapse. This effect has been observed among individuals who smoke (Curry, Marlatt, & Gordon, 1987; Kirchner, Shiffman, & Wileyto, 2012) and binge-eat (Grilo & Shiffman, 1994).

Handout 8.2, "Relapse Prevention," can help patients understand the difference between a lapse and a relapse as well as specific examples of how they might experience these different patterns. Once the patient understands this difference, the clinician can explain the nature of relapse and the importance of examining the cognitive processes that can cause a lapse to escalate into a relapse. At this point, it is usually most effective to ask patients to consider hypothetical examples that could apply to them. First, they are asked to consider examples of a lapse, and then to consider various scenarios that would lead from a lapse to relapse instead of a lapse leading to "back on track" status. The patient is then asked to consider specific situations that place him or her at risk of a lapse and potential relapse. The clinician can use examples of lapses and subsequent scenarios that have actually occurred during the course of therapy. The GOAL skill can be especially helpful when patients are faced with lapses and attempts to get back on track. As shown in the example below, short-term goals can include self-monitoring, CARE planning, and practicing skills.

Example Dialogue

CLINICIAN: As we get closer to the end of treatment we will want to start thinking about how to avoid lapses and relapses. Can you think of situations that you might continue to struggle with after treatment is over, situations where you might experience urges to binge-eat?

PATIENT: Realistically, I know I will still have days where I get upset after meetings with my boss.

CLINICIAN: In thinking about how to manage urges and possible lapses after treatment ends, sometimes the GOAL skill can be very helpful if you do end up struggling.

PATIENT: You mean setting goals not to binge?

CLINICIAN: Maybe, although the GOAL skill can be particularly useful in working toward doing something that will be helpful, rather than not doing something, like binge eating. For example, if you notice that you are having urges to binge and purge after your weekly meetings with your boss, you could try setting a goal to do something that would be helpful.

PATIENT: Oh, I get what you mean . . . like setting a goal to check in with myself about my feelings before and after the meeting. Usually the binges after those work meetings happen when I'm upset.

CLINICIAN: That's a great example. I'm wondering if it would be useful to define that goal in more specific behavioral terms, like where and when you could do that checking in?

PATIENT: Maybe to sit in my office and practice the FEEL skill for 10 minutes before and 10 minutes after each meeting. I think that might help, especially if my boss says something that upsets me.

CLINICIAN: That sounds like a very useful goal. It's also helpful to set up a target end date for the goal rather than implying that you will pursue it indefinitely. How long do you think you would keep doing the FEEL check-in when you have work meetings?

PATIENT: A month. I think that would feel manageable without feeling like I am committing to do it forever.

CLINICIAN: That sounds like an ideal goal, and one that would really help prevent binge eating and purging after those challenging meetings.

Particularly if self-evaluation and self-standards were a focus of Phase III, relapse can arise if the patient has unrealistic and rigid self-standards about recovery, especially the expectation that "success" means not encountering future struggles. If self-standards have been emphasized, the abstinence violation effect can be discussed in the context of modifying expectations to be more flexible and accepting. In fact, Marlatt (1996) found that the two most frequent precipitating events in relapse among alcoholics were negative emotional states and interpersonal conflict. Because self-discrepancy has been linked to negative affect, relapse may be less likely when patients continue to work on reducing their level of self-discrepancy after treatment ends. Likewise, self-regulatory behaviors and interpersonal problems are associated with affective states and therefore are likely to play a role in the maintenance of abstinence. Of particular importance is the maintenance of self-accepting behaviors after a lapse. Self-acceptance allows the realistic acknowledgment of a slip, which can then be seen as an opportunity for the patient to learn from it and get back on track. Maintaining self-acceptance is less likely to lead to negative affect, including self-criticism and guilt, which may be particularly associated with bulimic symptoms (Berg et al., 2013), and will reduce the risk of a lapse becoming a relapse.

Once high-risk situations and potential lapse and relapse scenarios are identified, specific plans should be designated for particular situations. Specific steps include resuming self-monitoring, creating CARE plans, completing a SEA Change Diary, and using ICAT-BN skills (e.g., FEEL, ACT, and GOAL), reaching out to friends and family for support, and/or contacting a clinician. As shown in Handout 8.3, "Lapse Plans," patients can review the use of specific skills as well as considering various lapse and relapse scenarios. The ICAT-BN skills should be emphasized, and specific plans for implementing them in response to potential lapses can be discussed. Handout 8.4, "Questions to Ask Yourself If You Have a Slip or a Lapse," is also useful for helping patients ask themselves questions in the context of a lapse, and Handout 8.5, "Toward a Healthy Lifestyle," can be particularly useful for facilitating ongoing skill practice and support seeking after treatment ends. Several years after her treatment ended, for example, Jackie (who was described in Chapter 1) discovered that her husband was having an affair with a younger woman. Convinced that her husband was no longer attracted to her because of her weight, she began restricting her food intake again in an attempt to be more attractive to her husband. At first she felt more in control because she was losing weight; however, after she found some explicit texts that her husband had received from this younger woman, Jackie had her first binge-eating and purging episode in years. After 3 days of binge eating and purging, Jackie reviewed the lapse and relapse plans she had created during her ICAT-BN treatment sessions. First, she created CARE plans for the following week and started self-monitoring her eating. She also used the FEEL skill to identify her intense feelings of anger and sadness. Although the intensity of her painful feelings was difficult to endure at first, she also realized that the more she could practice "sitting with" these emotions, the less she felt the urge to binge eat. She used the ACT skill to increase her self-soothing and self-distracting behaviors (e.g., taking walks, joined a book club) and scheduled a vacation for later in the month to visit a friend who lived out of state. Jackie decided that she would make an appointment for a booster session with her ICAT-BN clinician if she continued to binge-eat and purge after she returned from her vacation.

HEALTHY LIFESTYLE PLANNING

In our initial ICAT-BN pilot trials, healthy lifestyle planning was an aspect of treatment that was rated among the most helpful for our participants. As important as it is to educate about relapse prevention, healthy lifestyle planning emphasizes ways of continuing to recover from BN and, even more significantly, to create a meaningful life in the absence of the eating disorder. Handouts 8.5, "Toward a Healthy Lifestyle," and 8.6, "Healthy Lifestyle Plan," are typically assigned as homework in one of the last few sessions. The clinician can encourage the patient to step back and consider his or her day-to-day life, especially what makes it both healthy and meaningful, from a broader perspective. The clinician can emphasize to the patient that the "momentary" focus and planning skills important in ICAT-BN can also be used toward furthering positive behaviors that support and sustain self-care. Patients may also recognize that important activities that had been replaced by eating disorder behaviors may now be reintroduced. A lifestyle balancing pleasures and stressors is primary in preventing relapse (Marlatt & Gordon, 1985), and a lifestyle plan helps consolidate treatment progress. As shown in the following case example, identifying activities that used to be meaningful to the patient can be helpful in healthy lifestyle planning (see Figure 8.1).

Example Dialogue

CLINICIAN: So let's talk about what it was like to fill out your Healthy Lifestyle Plan.

PATIENT: It was kind of strange, because it reminded me of all the things that I used to do that I don't anymore. It made me realize how much time I spent binge eating and purging and obsessing about my weight and how much more time I have now.

CLINICIAN: What kinds of things did you used to do?

PATIENT: I really love animals and I used to volunteer at an animal shelter. I loved doing that. Also, I used to go to spiritual meetings every week with some of my closest friends. I haven't talked to any of them in a year.

Healthy Lifestyle Plan

Hours per Week	Describe Activities
40–45	Work/School *Some weeks I have to work more than 40 hours but I need to not work too much or else my exercise falls by the wayside and my mood gets worse.*
3	Physical activity *Lift weights 3 days a week for 30 minutes and do cardio 2 days a week for 45 minutes*
3.5 during the week 6 or more on weekends	Time alone, meditation, relaxation, spirituality *I'll practice mindfulness for 30 minutes before bedtime. On the weekends I will have at least 3 hours a day relaxing (versus doing chores/errands).*
2 on weekends, 1 during the week	Recreation, hobbies, cultural pursuits *On the weekends I'll spend at least 2 hours volunteering at an animal shelter. I will also start a weekly training program to become a foster parent for animals.*
1–2 hours a day	Relationships *I will work out with my friend at the gym once a week and spend time with my family and friends at night and on the weekends. I will make sure that I text a friend or family member at least once a day to avoid getting isolated again.*
None now	Therapy/Support *I'm going to see how I do without therapy but will contact my clinician if I need more support.*
6 hours	Meals (include grocery shopping and preparation of meals) *I'll shop on Sunday and prepare meals for the first part of the week. Wednesday I have a short day at work so I can prepare more meals then for the last days of the week. I'll bring lunches and snacks to work since I do better eating there rather than going out to eat.*
8 hours/night	Sleep *Sleep is really critical to my health, ideally 8 hours a night. I will plan to go to bed by 10 p.m. during the week and 11:30 on weekends.*

FIGURE 8.1. Example of a completed healthy lifestyle plan.

CLINICIAN: I am trying to read what you are feeling right now as you are talking about it.

PATIENT: A mix—sad that I haven't been doing those things, but excited to start again. I put them on my schedule. I even texted my friend who runs the spiritual group, and she said they all want me to start coming again. I haven't contacted the animal shelter yet because I want to check out a few online to see which is closest to where I live, but I plan to do that this week.

CLINICIAN: That sounds wonderful.

PATIENT: Filling out that plan also made me realize that I need to make sleep a priority. I never have, but when I get enough sleep, I feel better and have fewer urges to binge.

CLINICIAN: Yes, that's a really useful observation. You could even use the GOAL skill around changing your sleep patterns if you think it would be helpful.

TERMINATION AND ENDING TREATMENT

Typically confined to Phase IV and the final portion of treatment, termination emphasizes strategies to facilitate continued improvement as well as long-term self-care and a healthy lifestyle. Termination should be discussed before Phase IV begins so that the patient has time to become accustomed to the idea of treatment ending.

Clinicians and patients often wonder when treatment should end. The clearest reason to end ICAT-BN is that the patient never or rarely exhibits eating disorder behaviors. In addition, termination is indicated when the patient has a clear understanding about both the function that the eating disorder behaviors used to serve as well as healthy behavioral alternatives that are effective for coping with situations and emotions that have served as bulimic triggers. Often, patients will express readiness to stop treatment along with some sadness about the formal ending of the therapeutic relationship. Sometimes patients may be reluctant to end treatment and do not feel ready to be without the support of the clinician. In these cases, the patient and clinician should discuss whether the patient is primarily anxious about ending treatment but seems capable of making this transition or whether the patient should continue treatment to consolidate therapeutic gains. In addition, the clinician and the patient can collaborate to set a tapering schedule in which they meet increasingly less frequently (e.g., biweekly, and then monthly). Alternatively, booster sessions can be scheduled at the end of treatment for several months after termination (e.g., Fairburn, 2008). If the clinician is available, patients can be encouraged to call him or her after treatment is ended if they feel at risk of relapse and need professional support. Prior to the final session, the clinician should provide the patient with information about whom to contact in the case of relapse (specifically, whether the patient can recontact the clinician) and/or circumstances in which the patient can contact the clinician. Being explicit about the clinician's accessibility after treatment prior to the final session is especially important in facilitating honest discussions about the meaning of termination to both the patient and the clinician. The patient and clinician can also use termination as an opportunity to discuss whether adjunctive or alternative treatment would be beneficial (e.g., intensive treatment, couple counseling, and psychopharmacological interventions for depression).

Handout 8.7, "Finishing Treatment," can be given prior to the final treatment session and reviewed as part of the final session. The theme of the final session, even among patients who are still symptomatic, is a review of accomplishments and change. The final session also provides a last opportunity to discuss plans and ongoing improvement. Because ICAT-BN is emotion focused, the brevity of the termination phase should in no way limit the importance of attending to and discussing the patient's feelings about ending treatment. The range of feelings that patients may have in finishing is substantial, including grief/sadness, anger, relief, gratitude, and happiness. Being attuned to nonverbal emotional cues is especially critical in Phase IV; its importance can be seen in the following case example.

Example Dialogue

CLINICIAN: As we were talking about how the next session is our final session, I noticed that you were smiling but also, perhaps, tearful.

PATIENT: Well, yes. It's funny, because I do feel so happy about the progress I have made, and, honestly, getting to these sessions from work has been a real challenge. So I am kind of relieved that I won't be so worried about leaving work and the traffic. But I do feel so sad—like I wish I could keep seeing you even though I think I am ready to take a shot at doing this on my own.

CLINICIAN: Can you talk more about feeling sad?

PATIENT: Well, it's just that you understood me and I have never once felt ashamed with you about being bulimic. And that's so different because with everyone else, I am just so mortified. But from the beginning you have been so accepting of me, and even talked about how my bulimia might have been helpful with my feelings! I will miss seeing you and I will miss talking with you.

CLINICIAN: I am sad about our ending too. Your progress has been amazing. I am so thrilled to have been able to work with you, and I am especially grateful for your honesty with me because I know you have said how hard that was at first. I completely agree with you: You *are* ready to do this on your own. But I will miss you too.

SUMMARY

The final phase of ICAT-BN emphasizes the consolidation of treatment progress as well as strategies for preventing relapse. Specifically, Phase IV focuses on providing education about the difference between a lapse and a relapse, the value of monitoring impulses using the WAIT skill, and the benefits of establishing a healthy lifestyle plan. Because patients often have emotions associated with ending treatment, remaining attuned to feelings within and outside of sessions is especially important in Phase IV. In addition, treatment termination can include discussion about the need for further treatment, the possibility of scheduling follow-up "booster" sessions, and specific steps the patient can pursue in the event of relapse, including recontacting the clinician.

Part III

ICAT-BN PATIENT HANDOUTS AND SKILL CARDS

Patient Handouts

Understanding Bulimia Nervosa

Bulimia nervosa cannot be easily understood. Numerous factors have been suggested to play a role in its development, including dieting, concerns about weight, a family history of obesity or dieting, cultural or social pressure to lose weight, depression, family problems, low self-esteem, genetics, biological factors, and a history of childhood maltreatment. However, none of these issues is *necessarily* present for all people who develop bulimia nervosa. It is also unlikely that any one of these factors by itself will lead to the development of bulimia nervosa. Furthermore, some factors that may be involved in the development of bulimia nervosa may not be the same factors that make the behaviors continue once they start. For example, an individual may have bulimic symptoms, at least in part, as a result of dieting; however, the bulimic behavior may continue after the dieting ends because binge eating and purging help to reduce negative feelings, so it is hard to stop. Although what causes and maintains bulimia nervosa for a given person is highly complex, it is important for you to have some understanding of what factors may be involved in causing and maintaining bulimic symptoms. The theory that underlies ICAT is outlined in the accompanying figure and described below.

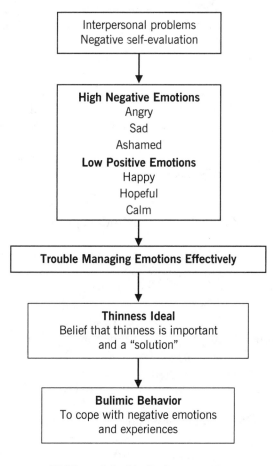

ICAT model of bulimia nervosa.

(continued)

Negative Self-Evaluation and Interpersonal Problems

People with bulimia nervosa often report difficulties in particular parts of their lives, including relationships with other people as well as harsh and critical evaluation of themselves. In ICAT, we believe that relationships and negative self-evaluation are important in the development of bulimia nervosa, particularly because these types of experiences (e.g., troublesome relationships and self-criticism) cause negative emotions and make it difficult to experience positive emotions. The types of relationship problems that are important in bulimia nervosa can vary substantially among people. Some individuals may get along fairly well with most people but have a lot of conflict with a small number of people, often family members. Other individuals might have great difficulty with intimate relationships, which leaves them feeling isolated. Other people might be characterized as extremely shy and withdrawn, which can lead them to feel lonely. Others might seem to get along well with virtually everybody they meet but have difficulties when they compare themselves to other people and feel inadequate or "not good enough."

Another common experience among people with bulimia nervosa is feeling that they don't live up to their own standards (i.e., "I am not good enough") and being extremely self-critical when they fail to live up to them. When people believe they have not lived up to their standards, they often work extremely hard to change. In bulimia nervosa, the experience of feeling like one is not meeting standards of appearance can lead to cutting back on eating, increasing exercise, or purging. However, these steps can make bulimic symptoms worse. Not all individuals with bulimia are extremely self-critical. Some are very self-controlling and try to make sure that nothing ever goes wrong. Some of these individuals also have high standards for themselves. Others are not very attentive to themselves and drift into risky or problematic situations, which they later regret. Sometimes this might be situations with food that lead to more bulimic behavior. An important common theme among relationship problems, negative self-evaluation, self-criticism, and self-neglect is that these experiences lead to negative emotions, which then ultimately lead to decisions that result in binge eating and purging or other types of bulimic behaviors.

Emotions and Their Management

Painful emotions or feelings are often difficult for people with bulimia nervosa to tolerate. Some people feel overwhelmed by emotions and are unsure how to cope with them. Others feel out of touch with their emotions and are not sure what they are experiencing. *Experiencing and understanding your emotions is extremely important to your recovery.* Emotions are a natural part of living and help us to realize what is important; they also motivate us to take action. There are six primary emotions: joy, sadness, fear, anger, disgust, and surprise. Other primary emotions may include contempt, guilt, interest, and shame. When you experience these emotions, you will notice particular physical sensations, facial expressions, and motivations to take action. These emotions indicate that something important is happening. This is why it is important to learn to pay attention to them. Emotions can be very difficult to identify and express but critically important to understanding and changing your bulimic patterns.

This treatment is designed to help people with bulimia nervosa identify more clearly what they are feeling and to make healthy choices in response to these feelings. Negative feelings are a natural part of being human and cannot be avoided. Positive feelings are also an essential part of being human and should be experienced fully. Many people with bulimia nervosa engage in bulimic or other problematic behaviors when they are experiencing strong emotions. Bulimic behaviors may actually help manage strong emotions. One of the most important parts of this treatment is to understand that when you are feeling strong emotions it is *extremely important to identify healthy action choices.*

(continued)

The Thinness Ideal and Dieting

In our culture, it is understandable to believe that if we look attractive, particularly in terms of body size and shape, we will feel good about ourselves and be admired by others. Our culture is full of media images of attractive people, typically thin or even underweight, looking happy, receiving admiration, and appearing to be in control of their lives. Despite the fact that these media images are unrealistic and often generated or altered by computers, many people are strongly influenced by these cultural messages. They believe that they have to be thin to be attractive, well liked, and successful. People who believe this are often more likely to develop bulimia nervosa, in part due to the difference between how they actually view themselves (their actual self) and how they want to be (their desired self). Their pursuit of thinness as a "solution" to their dissatisfaction comes with the risks of dietary restriction and purging. Because dietary restriction and purging increase the risk of binge eating, this pattern often leads to a self-destructive cycle of bulimic behavior.

Binge Eating, Purging, and Other Bulimic Behaviors

Why might a person who is quite concerned about thinness and body shape engage in binge eating? In this treatment, we believe that binge-eating episodes tend to occur for two primary reasons. First, in order to influence their shape and weight, individuals often limit the types and amount of food they eat to such an extent that they trigger binge eating. For this reason, this treatment focuses on ensuring that you eat sufficient food to prevent nutritional deprivation and binge eating. Second, binge eating might be a means of reducing feelings like sadness, guilt, or shame, while increasing contentment or calmness. Most people with bulimia understand that binge eating is not a permanent solution to their problems, but it has become a way of dealing with feelings and issues in their lives.

Purging in the form of vomiting tends to follow binge episodes and may also help with negative feelings, particularly fears of gaining weight after a binge-eating episode. Using laxatives may also give individuals some reassurance that even though they are binge eating they can control their weight. Similarly, diet pills and water pills may help people with bulimia believe that they have some ability to control the negative effects of binge eating as well as to control their weight and appearance. In fact, none of these purging techniques is effective for long-term weight control, and they often have extremely harmful health effects.

It might be useful to think about what factors contribute to your binge eating and purging. What role does binge eating and purging serve in your life? Has your bulimic behavior become important as a way of dealing with situations and experiences in your life? Understanding more fully the role that bulimic behaviors have come to serve in your life can help you to change the patterns.

An Example of Emotions, Coping, and Bulimia Nervosa

Self-evaluation, negative feelings, and coping choices can be important in causing and maintaining bulimic behavior. Consider Jenny:

> Jenny described herself as "not good at anything." She believed that she was not living up to the standard she was holding for herself and felt inadequate. Although many of her friends thought she was happy, she had secret feelings of shame and dissatisfaction with herself. She also secretly felt competitive with her friends about appearance and attractiveness. She began to think that if she were thinner and more attractive (her desired self), "everything would be okay." Jenny tried many things to attain her desired self. For example, she became perfectionistic about her schoolwork and her eating habits. She strictly limited her carbohydrate, fat, and caloric intake. She also found herself allowing others to tell

(continued)

161

her what to do and how to behave in hopes of getting others to like and accept her. The fact that she only lost a small amount of weight after changing her eating habits led to her to pursue more restrictive dieting. As a result of her submissive interpersonal patterns she began to feel frustrated in her relationships, complaining that others took advantage of her. She began to feel that she couldn't trust anyone. The combination of undernourishment from dieting and interpersonal distress from her submissive patterns led her to feel increasingly unhappy. She began to have binge-eating episodes followed by self-induced vomiting because of her fear that binge eating would lead to weight gain. These bulimic episodes became more frequent, and she had a sense of losing control over her eating entirely. When she would binge-eat, she described experiencing a sense of relief from the pressure of dieting and trying to control her eating, almost as if she was on a mental "vacation." She was also extremely upset by her loss of control and viewed her vomiting as a way to quickly try to "clean the slate" and regain self-control.

As illustrated by this example, several factors seem to be important in the development of Jenny's bulimia nervosa. First, there was a difference between the way she perceived herself and the way she wished to be (particularly regarding her physical appearance), leading her to believe that she was not good enough. Second, this belief that she was inadequate was associated with feeling "upset." Third, she developed self-destructive *ways of relating to herself* and *ways of relating to other people,* which were an effort to attain her desired self. Part of her attempt to cope with her feelings was her decision to *diet,* and because nutritional deprivation made it difficult for her to maintain her strict diet, she felt even more distress. Dieting and distress combined to increase her risk of binge eating and purging. Once this pattern began, she found it difficult to stop. Jenny's problem helps us to see how bulimia nervosa is a complex issue that involves more than just food and eating. Each of these areas—your self-evaluation, your feelings, and the way you cope with others, yourself, and your eating patterns—will be a focus of your treatment.

Overview of Treatment

This treatment is primarily focused on four major goals. Each goal is described below.

1. Realistic Self-Evaluation and Improved Relationships

Treatment will focus on helping you to identify how you *actually* perceive yourself and how this may differ from how you *desire* or expect to be. We think it is important for you to gain an accurate and complete picture of yourself, your talents, abilities, and appearance. Frequently, people with bulimia nervosa maintain an inaccurately negative view of themselves, and they do not recognize their positive features. Additionally, we will encourage you to examine the standards you use to evaluate yourself. Individuals with bulimia frequently choose extremely high standards that are difficult to attain. In spite of their efforts, individuals with bulimia may never reach their standards, which is disappointing. These self-standards may include appearance as well as other aspects of themselves. In this treatment, we will help you identify flexible and reasonable standards to pursue.

It will be important for you to think about how relationships relate to your bulimic behavior. Relationship problems seem to be a common trigger for emotional stress and bulimic behavior. Do you find yourself in relationships or social situations that seem to set you up for bulimic behavior? What is it about those situations that makes them so difficult? Is this a relationship that you might be able to change? If not, can you learn to tolerate the relationship or accept the limitations inherent in the relationship? What skills might help you to manage this relationship more effectively? These are important questions for you to think about in your treatment. Having healthy, adaptive relationships is likely to be an important part of your recovery.

2. Normal Eating

The early phases of treatment will help you think about ways to eat more normally to support your health and self-care. Evidence suggests that people with bulimia nervosa eat food in a way that is nutritionally unhealthy. Most often, the pattern shifts between dieting and binge eating. Food restriction is a trigger for binge eating. For a variety of physical and psychological reasons, developing a pattern of eating that includes an adequate amount of food and a variety of foods eaten in planned meals and snacks will help you recover. We will encourage you to try to develop a schedule of planned meals and snacks to support your health and reduce the chance of binge eating.

Until you are eating sufficient meals and snacks, it will be difficult to know if your binge eating is a response to not eating enough or if it is the result of interpersonal or emotional factors. Therefore, we recommend that you work on giving up dieting and food restriction and start to eat adequate amounts of food early in treatment. You will be supported in numerous ways as you attempt to accomplish this task, including learning alternative coping strategies. *This treatment encourages maintaining a healthy body weight and does not promote weight gain beyond that level. It also does not promote weight loss.*

(continued)

3. Experiencing Emotional States and Understanding Cues

We encourage you to begin to pay attention to the emotions you experience. In this treatment, dieting and bulimic behavior are thought to be used as a way to cope with unpleasant feelings. Bulimic behavior may help you temporarily avoid negative feelings by increasing your focus on aspects of the eating disorder, such as dieting or distraction through binge eating and purging.

We believe that experiencing a wide range of feelings, both positive and negative, is a normal part of life. Therefore, in this therapy you will be encouraged to be sensitive to your emotions as they occur and to try to "stick with them." Also, it will be important to understand the overall meaning of the feeling. What is the significance of the feeling in your life? From the beginning to the end of your treatment, your clinician will be very attentive to your feelings during sessions, as well as checking in with you about the feelings you experience in between sessions. We encourage you to discuss these feelings as openly as possible, although we recognize that this may be difficult at first.

In your treatment, we will also help you to become more aware of cues for your emotional distress and your bulimic behavior. As you become more aware of your feelings, it will be important to try to identify situations or experiences that trigger those emotions. These could involve relationships, self-evaluation, the way you treat yourself, or even being in difficult food-related situations. Nonetheless, learning about cues in your world that are associated with risks for bulimic behavior is extremely important to your recovery.

4. Managing Your Bulimic Urges

It's important to find adaptive strategies for managing your urge to engage in bulimic behavior. As we have suggested, bulimic urges may be triggered by significant food restriction or emotions and stress. It is also important to consider the possibility that urges may be triggered by boredom or an absence of positive feelings. Regardless of the emotions you encounter, you can develop skills to manage those moments without turning to bingeing, purging, or other eating disorder behaviors. We encourage you to use the skills that we introduce in ICAT to help you through these moments. A fundamental idea in this treatment is to find a healthy substitute for what the bulimic behavior gives you. Is it distraction, comfort, or simple relief from stress? You will want to talk with your clinician about how your bulimic behavior might be helping you as well as more adaptive ways to take care of these needs.

Thinking about How These Issues Affect You Every Day

Words like *emotion* and *self-evaluation* are not simply clinical terms that we use to understand bulimia nervosa. Rather, these are words that can capture important moments that occur in your everyday life. If you believe that you are not good enough, there may be moments when you feel that you are not living up to the standards you hold for yourself. When that occurs, it is likely that you will feel some kind of negative emotion. As this is happening, you will make choices about what you are going to do about these negative feelings. It is these moments that may ultimately lead to binge eating and purging. For example, your standard for yourself may be to have excellent job performance. If something then goes wrong at work, you may feel badly about yourself. These negative emotions may then contribute to binge eating and purging. At these particular moments, binge eating might feel helpful. It may distract you and help you feel calm. Unfortunately, these benefits do not last, and people who binge-eat often find that the short-term "positive" effects don't last and ultimately they feel worse.

(continued)

As you stop your bulimic behaviors, you may notice some changes. You may become more aware of your negative feelings because you are not using your old coping strategies to avoid them. As part of your therapy, your clinician will work with you to find different ways to meet the need previously met by your bulimic behavior. Your bulimic behavior has developed as a way to cope with problems. As part of your recovery, please continue to try to identify these problems and work with your therapist to develop new strategies to help you to deal with these problems more effectively.

HANDOUT 5.3

Preparing for Treatment

Most people who seek help for bulimia nervosa have had symptoms of the disorder for quite a while, often years. There are typically several reasons why treatment isn't sought right away. Sometimes people don't know where to find help or can't afford it, or it simply isn't available where they live. Sometimes, people feel embarrassed about their bulimic symptoms and are afraid to seek help. Another reason is that they can see both advantages and disadvantages to stopping the bulimic symptoms.

By the time someone seeks help, there are typically a number of problems caused by the bulimic symptoms. Physical, emotional, financial, social, occupational, and relationship problems often occur. At the same time, stopping the bulimic behaviors can be frightening. The symptoms may seem to help you to deal with painful emotions or make you feel thinner. These positive aspects of the bulimic behaviors can make them hard to give up. Specific fears—especially the fear of gaining weight—can also keep people from changing their bulimic behaviors.

When starting treatment, the advantages of changing eating behaviors usually are greater than the disadvantages—sometimes a lot greater and sometimes only a little greater. No matter what the balance, it's important to recognize that there are both positive and negative aspects of your bulimic behaviors.

Below are some questions to begin to think about as you start treatment. Please write down your responses below to share with your therapist.

1. Can you identify any problems associated with your eating disorder? Please describe them.

_____

_____

_____

2. Why do you want to change your eating disorder behaviors?

_____

_____

_____

3. What are the positive aspects of your eating disorder? How has it benefited or helped you? Are there reasons you do NOT want to change?

_____

_____

_____

4. Are there things about your eating disorder or its consequences that have begun to worry you or concern you?

_____

_____

_____

(continued)

5. What have other people told you about your eating disorder? Are other people worried?

_____

_____

_____

6. If you continue your eating disorder behaviors, what effect will it have on your life in 5 years? In 10 years? When you imagine your life at that time, do you imagine your eating disorder as a part of it?

_____

_____

_____

7. What are the most important things that make you think you need to make a change in your eating patterns?

_____

_____

_____

8. On the following scale, mark with an X the box that best describes your attitude about changing your *binge eating*:

I don't see a need to change.	I think about change but don't really think I need to do it.	I need to change but am really afraid to try.	I know I need to change and am planning to do it.	I am ready to change now.
☐	☐	☐	☐	☐

9. On the following scale mark with an X the box that best describes your attitude about changing your *purging* (e.g., vomiting, laxatives, diet pills, diuretics/water pills):

I don't see a need to change.	I think about change but don't really think I need to do it.	I need to change but am really afraid to try.	I know I need to change and am planning to do it.	I am ready to change now.
☐	☐	☐	☐	☐

10. On the following scale mark with an X the box that best describes your attitude about changing your *dieting or food restriction patterns*:

I don't see a need to change.	I think about change but don't really think I need to do it.	I need to change but am really afraid to try.	I know I need to change and am planning to do it.	I am ready to change now.
☐	☐	☐	☐	☐

Beginning to Notice My Feelings

On this page, you will see pictures of faces showing a number of feelings that humans experience. It may be helpful for you to look through these different faces and feelings to learn about the variety of emotions that you may have.

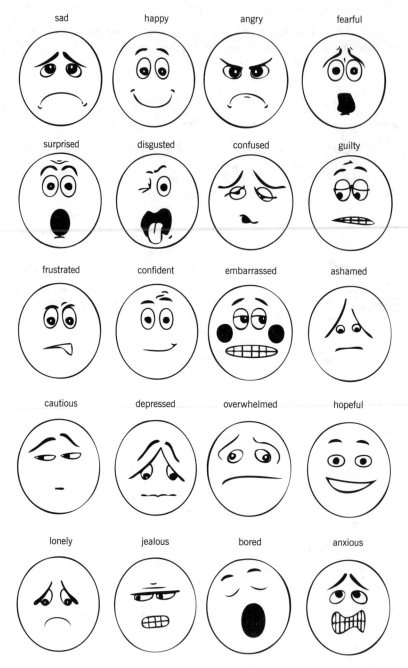

The FEEL Skill

In ICAT, we have identified a series of skills to help you recover. The first is the FEEL skill, which is designed to help you identify and experience your emotions more fully. Emotions are a natural part of living, and learning to fully experience both negative and positive feelings is a basic skill that is part of being a healthy person. The FEEL skill is essential in helping you feel more comfortable with your emotions and giving you a sense of greater control and flexibility in your life. Below are the steps of the FEEL skill. Practice it twice a day (ideally 10–15 minutes at a time). Sometimes using the FEEL skill will be easy, sometimes not. As you practice, you will be able to identify and label your feelings more accurately.

Focus	• Find a quiet place. • Let yourself sit for a minute. • Pay attention to your body sensations. • Try not to judge or evaluate yourself.
Experience	• Allow a feeling to come. • You may not know what to call it. • Pay attention to the feeling. • Practice staying with it for a while. • Notice how your body is feeling.
Examine	• Start to wonder what this is. • What do you think this feeling is about? • Where is it coming from?
Label	• Can you give it a name? • Try the name out. Does it fit? • Is that all of it, or is there another feeling? If yes, repeat.

Why Write Down What You Eat?

Now that you are starting treatment, it will be important for you and your therapist to learn about the details of your eating patterns, your feelings, and your behaviors. Starting now, we will ask you to write down *everything* that you eat, along with any symptoms you have and any physical activities you do. Writing down what you eat can be very challenging but it is important to do for several reasons:

1. Writing a detailed list of what you eat and how you are feeling will help you and your therapist figure out what is working as well as what happens when you are struggling. Your food record will give you and your therapist a very clear picture of what you are eating, how you are feeling, and what you are doing. You and your therapist will use this information to guide your treatment.

2. Writing down what you eat will help you be more aware of what you are eating and how you are feeling. The more aware you are of your eating and your feelings, the more you will be able to change them.

3. Writing down what you eat has been found in research to be helpful in changing bulimic symptoms, and many people describe it as a useful part of their recovery.

For your recording sheet to work, *make sure to write down what you have eaten as soon as possible after you have eaten it.* It helps to write down what you drink as well, although you do not have to record every sip of water. Many people are embarrassed about writing down their binge-eating episodes and sharing this information with their therapist. If you are concerned about what your therapist might think, please share your feelings with your therapist so that you can be reassured that writing down what you eat, including your binge-eating episodes, is a safe and helpful step in changing your patterns.

Some people who start writing down what they eat find that at first this process is quite challenging. It can be hard to remember to write things down immediately after eating. Some people find that when they start writing down what they are eating, they spend more time thinking about their eating. Although having this kind of awareness will be very important, it can be hard at first. Others find that the process of writing down what they are eating brings up strong feelings. Be sure to talk about these feelings with your therapist and to write them down on your record. *Most people find that writing down what they eat and how they are feeling becomes much more comfortable after a week or two of practice.*

Daily Food Record

Date _____

Time	Type* (M, S, R, V, L, D, E, B)	Food/Beverage	Notes (location, feelings)
Exercise (Type, Duration):			

*Type: M = meal; S = snack; R = restricting; V = vomiting; L= laxative; D= diuretic; E = exercise; B = binge/overeating/eating more than planned/loss of control.

Sample Completed Daily Food Record

Date _____

Time	Type* (M, S, R, V, L, D, E, B)	Food/Beverage	Notes (location, feelings)
7:00	M, R	½ bagel, plain Water (1 bottle)	Breakfast at home Feeling fat, trying to cut back
10:00		Coffee (1 cup)	Work, stressed about meeting
12:00	M, R	Salad (2 cups) Water (1 bottle)	At work, preparing for meeting; Feeling worried about meeting; Trying not to eat much, skipped salad dressing
2:30	S, R	Nonfat yogurt (1/2 cup)	Worried about meeting; Saw cookies in the break room; Had yogurt instead of cookies
3:00	S	2 cookies (chocolate chip)	Ate during meeting; Unhappy about meeting; Mad at myself for not doing a better presentation
3:30	B	5 cookies (chocolate chip)	Can't stop eating; mad, sad
5:30	B	3 cheeseburgers; Fries (5 cups); Milkshake (1 large)	Stopped at drive-through; Eating out of control; Upset but can't stop; Have to purge, scared of weight
5:45	V		Stopped at store; might as well keep eating; feel disgusted with myself; feel fat
6:00	B	Cookies (sandwich), 1 pkg; Ice cream, (2 pints)	
6:30	V		Feel gross, sad, mad
9:00		Water (1 bottle)	Tired, going to bed
Exercise (Type, Duration):	None		

*Type: M = meal; S = snack; R = restricting; V = vomiting; L= laxative; D= diuretic; E = exercise; B = binge/overeating/eating more than planned/loss of control.

Why Eat Regular Meals and Snacks?

People who binge-eat often restrict food intake by dieting, following eating "rules," and avoiding certain foods in order to impact their weight and shape or avoid binge eating; however, food restriction can actually *cause* binge eating. The best example of the risks of food restriction is based on research conducted at the University of Minnesota in the 1940s in order to determine how to best help prisoners of war from World War II. The study was trying to understand the effects of food restriction and the process of weight restoration following semistarvation among healthy adult men with no history of eating problems. Subjects in this study were placed on low-calorie diets to induce weight loss. After a period of time, the men began to exhibit many *symptoms of semistarvation*:

- Mood problems (e.g., anxiety, depression, and irritability)
- Thinking constantly about food
- Feeling cold all the time
- Concentration problems
- Loss of interest and pleasure in things they used to enjoy

One of the most important findings was what happened when these men were allowed to eat normally again: *many men experienced binge-eating episodes in which they uncontrollably ate large amounts of food*. Some men ended up gaining weight above their original predieting weight. After returning to their normal eating habits, the men eventually stopped binge eating and stabilized at their previous body weight.

The results of this study suggest that *binge eating may be a "natural" response to not eating enough* and may have evolved in humans as self-protection when food was scarce. Dieting and food restriction may "trick" our body into believing that there is a food shortage, resulting in binge eating. There is also evidence that dieting slows metabolism, making weight gain more likely.

Another set of studies indicates that dieting poses psychological as well as biological risks. Research on dieting has found that when individuals deprive themselves of "forbidden" foods (usually high in sugar or fat), they are more likely to overeat these foods when they are eventually exposed to them.

Individuals with bulimic symptoms often engage in a vicious cycle in which they try to control or restrict their food intake, binge-eat, then self-induce vomiting or use laxatives to try to prevent weight gain. An important fact to be aware of is that *self-induced vomiting does not rid the body of all the food eaten during a binge episode*. Research studies have found that only 50–70% of food consumed during binge-eating episodes is eliminated with self-induced vomiting. This finding means that 30–50% of the calories eaten during binge eating are retained in your body: In other words, much of what you eat during a binge episode actually stays inside of you.

Some people with bulimic symptoms take laxatives and diuretics (water pills). Laxatives and diuretics only serve to dehydrate the body by getting rid of fluid and don't really "get rid" of food.

We know that one of the main reasons people with bulimic symptoms purge using vomiting, laxatives, and diuretics is that they believe purging effectively "gets rid of" food they have eaten. Many people find that once they have made the decision to purge, they will actually eat more food, which makes the binge–purge cycle worse.

(continued)

What do these research findings tell us about changing bulimic eating patterns?

1. Restricting what you eat, dieting, and fasting can actually make binge eating worse: if you haven't eaten enough, you are at risk of binge eating.

2. Purging by self-induced vomiting, laxatives, or diuretics actually makes binge eating worse and it does not work to "get rid" of the food consumed during binge episodes.

3. Following a meal plan to help you figure out what, how much, and when to eat is essential to prevent binge eating and help you feel more control.

One of the most important things you can do to break the bulimic cycle is to start eating regular meals and snacks. We recognize that this process is very challenging, in part because of the fear that you might gain weight. Research suggests that most individuals recovering from bulimia nervosa who are within a healthy weight range do not end up gaining weight when they eat healthy amounts of varied foods for regular meals and snacks. Weight gain is less likely because eating enough food will prevent you from having binge-eating episodes (and, as described above, a percentage of what you eat is actually retained in the body). However, you may notice some temporary fluctuations as your body adjusts to eating normally.

The CARE Skill

At this point in treatment, you will start working on eating regular meals and snacks that include a variety of foods. Eating in a planned and structured manner will be a powerful way to stop your binge eating and is an important step toward caring for yourself.

Calmly	• Use the FEEL skill to get ready to CARE. • Find a quiet place that will help you remain calm.
Arrange	• Work on your meal plan at least a day ahead of time. • Take time to plan what, when, and where you will eat. • Avoid eating anything that you haven't planned to eat. • Devote time each day to work on and follow your meal plan.
Regular	• Eat regular meals and snacks to help prevent binge eating. • Try to get into a routine with your eating. • Follow your meal plan as closely as possible.
Eating	• Understand that eating is an important part of your self-care. • Check in with yourself about how you are feeling before, during, and after eating. • Try to allow yourself to eat a variety of food. • Experiment with eating differently.

To follow the CARE steps, your therapist will work with you to start planning your meals and snacks. It is important that you begin to eat regularly throughout the day, eat a variety of food, and gradually start to eat foods that you might have been avoiding in order to break the bulimic cycle.

You will continue to write down everything you eat as well as recording any bulimic symptoms you might have as part of the CARE skill. This process, along with planning what you will eat, is absolutely essential for your recovery in order to monitor your progress and become aware of your patterns and feelings. Your food records will help you and your therapist figure out how you can use the CARE skill most effectively.

(continued)

The CARE Skill: Calmly Arrange Regular Eating

Calmly   You may have a variety of feelings about changing your eating patterns. It is important to check in with yourself about what you are feeling and to discuss these feelings with your therapist. Try to work on your eating plans when you are calm and focused. It is important to make plans about your eating when you are not agitated, upset, or angry. Similarly, try to approach eating meals and snacks as calmly as possible. You may need to take a few moments to calm yourself down prior to eating.

Arrange   One of the most critical steps in changing your eating patterns is to *plan* your meals and snacks ahead of time and to follow your plan as closely as possible. Using the "arrange" step of CARE will help you eat thoughtfully and will serve as a basis of your self-care. Following the CARE steps will help you avoid "spur of the moment" decisions about what and when to eat, which can lead to binge eating, skipping meals, and out-of-control eating.

Regular   Planning and eating regular meals and snacks is a crucial part of changing your eating patterns. Skipping meals and snacks will put you at risk of binge eating because you will be food deprived and more likely to overeat when you do allow yourself to eat. Planning your meals and snacks will help you eat frequently enough to prevent these types of eating episodes from occurring.

Eating   Eating regular meals and snacks by following a meal plan will help prevent your binge eating and will also help your body "relearn" hunger and fullness. Over time, you may be able to follow these hunger and fullness "cues" in your body to decide when to start and stop eating. However, because these hunger and fullness cues don't work very well in people who are binge eating, following your meal plan will be the most effective way of deciding what to eat and when to start and stop eating in the early stages of treatment.

CARE Form

Now that you are planning what you eat ahead of time, you will use a different Daily Food Record form called the CARE form that includes a column for planning and a column to write down what you actually ate (if different from what you planned) as well as feelings and other information. *It is still very important that you write down what you eat as soon as possible after eating.* The CARE form allows you to use one sheet for both your planning and your recording. The plan is written on the left and the actual food eaten is written on the right. A sample completed CARE form with the meal plan and food record is shown in Handout 6.4.

Date _____

PLAN		ACTUAL		
Time	**Food/Drink**	**On plan (X) or "actual"**	**Type* (M, S, B, V, L, D, R, E)**	**Notes (feelings, skills used)**
Exercise (Type, duration):				

*Type: M = meal; S = snack; B = binge/overeating/eating more than planned/loss of control; V = vomiting; L = laxative; D = diuretic; R = restricting; E = exercise.

Sample Completed CARE Form

Date _____

	PLAN		ACTUAL	
Time	**Food/Drink**	**On plan (X) or "actual"**	**Type* (M, S, B, V, L, D, R, E)**	**Notes (feelings, skills used)**
8:00 am	½ Bagel w/peanut butter (1 T) + butter (1 T), coffee (1 C), yogurt (1 C), 1 orange	X	M	At home, late for work
12:00 pm	Tuna and cheese sandwich, salad with dressing	X	M	At work, lunch meeting
3:00 pm	Banana milkshake, pretzels	Actual: nothing		Skipped snack— busy Worked late
6:00 pm	Pasta (1 cup) with chicken, Marinara sauce, and cheese; salad with dressing; small brownie	Actual: 8:00 pm Cereal (10 cups), Ice Cream (2 pts), Chips (family-size bag)	B	Got home late, upset, tried to eat snack but ended up bingeing
8:00 pm	Cereal (1 cup) with cranberries and nuts	Actual: 9:00 pm Milk (3 cups)	V	Feel full, sad, fat

Exercise (Type, duration):   None

*Type: M = meal; S = snack; B = binge/overeating/eating more than planned/loss of control; V = vomiting; L = laxative; D = diuretic; R = restricting; E = exercise.

Meal Planning Using the CARE Skill

- Eat **three planned meals** a day (breakfast, lunch, and dinner) and several planned snacks each day. *Eating each morning is essential to prevent binge eating, even if you are not hungry and don't feel like eating.*

- **Avoid long breaks** between times that you eat your planned meals and snacks. Eating frequently enough is critical to prevent binge eating. We suggest eating a planned meal or snack every 2–3 hours.

- Eat a **variety** of foods. Variety is helpful to ensure adequate nutritional intake. Many people who struggle with bulimic patterns decide that certain foods are "bad" or "off limits" (usually foods that are high in fat, sugar, or carbohydrates) and don't allow themselves to eat these foods outside of binge-eating episodes. In fact, no foods are "bad" and it is okay to eat all foods in moderation. Many people who binge-eat often find that once they allow themselves to eat foods they like without feeling guilty or believing that a "rule" has been "broken," they are much less likely to have binge-eating episodes. However, you may have to start eating some of these foods that you have been avoiding more gradually. We encourage you to eat foods that might bring on strong feelings and then to use the FEEL skill to practice tolerating and understanding these feelings. Because limiting what you eat too much or too strictly can trigger binge eating, it is essential to eat foods that you enjoy in a planful way (e.g., eating planned desserts). Eating with self-care as your guide will help you learn how fulfilling, nutrient-rich, and good-tasting food consumed in appropriate portions makes you feel better physically and emotionally.

- **Follow your eating plan as closely as possible,** but allow yourself some *flexibility.* Many people with binge-eating problems find that they become preoccupied with counting calories, fat grams, or carbohydrates. The purpose of meal planning is to give you specific but flexible guidelines about what to eat to make sure you are getting adequate nutrition, to prevent binge eating, and to practice self-care. It is important to use these guidelines to help you, rather than viewing them as a new set of "rules" to follow strictly. For example, if an unplanned event occurs that interferes with your eating plan, it is okay to adjust your plan for the day in order to accommodate last-minute changes (e.g., you were planning to go out to lunch with a friend and he or she cancels).

- Make sure to **write down everything you eat** on your recording sheet, as soon as possible after eating (or check the column on the self-monitoring form if you ate everything according to your plan). You should write down meals, snacks, and binge-eating episodes. It can be hard to write these things down, but it will be extremely helpful. Also, make sure to note any binge-eating episodes and exercise on your recording sheet. When binge eating occurs, writing this down will help you learn how to prevent it in the future. It is also *very* important to *write down any emotions* you experience before, during, or after eating (you can use the back of your CARE record to write down your feelings if you need more space).

- Spend **time each day** writing out and reviewing your meal plan. Make sure to plan your meals and snacks the night before at the latest. Some people prefer to write out a weekly menu in order to purchase and prepare food ahead of time. Others prefer to write out their plan the night before when they have a clearer sense of their schedule. Some people find that they become more focused on food and eating when they are planning their eating, especially at first. Most people find that planning becomes **easier with practice.**

(continued)

- Some people wonder why they should eat when they are not hungry when following their meal plan and whether this "trains" the body to eat all of the time. In fact, **following your meal plan will help you regain (or develop) accurate experiences of hunger and fullness.** Because binge-eating behaviors interrupt the body's ability to experience hunger and fullness, they are not reliable "cues" early in treatment to determine when and what to eat. Instead, following your plan and eating according to the clock will help prevent binge-eating episodes. Eventually, as your eating patterns improve, you may notice that your body's hunger and fullness cues are more accurate and you can use them to help guide when and what you eat. Managing your hunger will also help you eat high-risk "binge foods" in reasonable amounts without experiencing a sense of loss of control. In the long term, the goal is to eat a variety of food without being afraid or feeling out of control, and to stop eating when you are satisfied, as well as to eat sufficient amounts of food to prevent binge eating and food preoccupation.

- Pay attention to **environmental factors that can trigger binge eating,** especially watching television, eating in restaurants, and keeping binge foods in your home and workplace. You may find it easier to eat your planned meals and snacks in environments that do not trigger binge eating, especially early in treatment. Later in treatment, you can practice eating in environments that might bring on strong feelings or urges to binge.

- Experiment with eating different types and amounts of food to see what works best for you. For example, you may find that you feel better if you eat a breakfast that includes protein (e.g., peanut butter instead of butter on toast). Try foods that you would not typically eat to see how they taste and how they make you feel. For example, do certain foods seem to give you energy? Do other foods seem to make you feel too full or sluggish? Keep notes on your CARE Form about what you learn.

- Many people find that the **anticipation of eating something that looks or smells appetizing can trigger binge eating.** Recent research suggests that some people who binge-eat might actually find the anticipation, or planning, of eating more rewarding than actually eating. Others find that eating food that tastes good to them is so rewarding they cannot stop eating once they start. If you find that the sight or smell of food triggers binge eating for you, be thoughtful about what food you keep in the house and how things like advertisements, being in restaurants, and shopping in grocery stores make you feel. You may find it helpful to avoid certain situations (leave the room during food commercials on television, drive a different way home from work to avoid seeing a certain restaurant, etc.) and to remind yourself that your brain is responding to food even if your body does not "need" to eat. Research suggests that certain people may be more sensitive to these types of food cues. If you respond strongly to the sight, smell, or thought of eating food, it is important for you to understand that this pattern does not mean you are weak or lack self-control. Instead, be gentle and treat yourself with self-care to support yourself in changing your patterns. Also, make sure the food you do eat tastes good and is rewarding to you, and that you eat food you enjoy in "safe" situations in which you are less likely to binge (e.g., ordering a slice of cake at a restaurant rather than keeping an entire cake at home).

Sample Menus for CARE Plans

Overview

One of the most important factors in selecting foods for your CARE plan is preference. To start, think about foods you eat regularly that you find satisfying and make you feel comfortable when you eat them (you may or may not be able to identify these types of foods). These foods can be incorporated as "regulars" into your CARE plan. For example, do you like oatmeal for breakfast? Fruit as a snack? Next, identify foods that might feel "risky" because they make you feel too full or you have overeaten them. Are there any that you could eat in small amounts in a planned manner when you are with other people (e.g., in a restaurant or at a friend's house for dinner)? If it feels too risky as far as triggering a binge-eating episode or purging, you can leave those off of your CARE plan for now, but you can experiment with introducing them later on. If you think you can eat some of your higher-risk foods, try including them in your meal plan in situations or at times of day that are "safe" (e.g., an ice-cream cone with friends as an afternoon snack).

Your clinician can also be helpful in coming up with ideas for your CARE plan. Websites and apps can provide food, menu, and meal planning ideas as well (e.g., *ChooseMyPlate.gov*; *www.choosemyplate.gov/healthy-eating-tips/sample-menus-recipes.html*). However, given that Internet information can be inaccurate and, at times, unhealthy in supporting your recovery (e.g., recommendations of inadequate energy intake), you will want to collaborate closely with your clinician to ensure that you are eating enough food.

Menu suggestions below are modified from *ChooseMyPlate.gov*; daily amounts shown in the menus below may be inadequate for individuals with moderate-to-high activity levels.

Menu #1

Breakfast
　Breakfast burrito
　　1 flour tortilla (7-inch diameter)
　　1 scrambled egg (with 1 teaspoon margarine)
　　1/3 cup black beans
　　2 tablespoons salsa
　1 cup orange juice
　1 cup skim milk

Lunch
　Roast beef sandwich
　　1 wheat sandwich bun
　　3 oz. lean roast beef
　　2 slices tomato
　　1/4 cup romaine lettuce
　　1/8 cup sautéed mushrooms (in 1 teaspoon oil)
　　1 1/2 oz. mozzarella cheese
　　1 teaspoon mustard
　Small bag of potato chips

Snack
　1 piece fruit (or 1 cup fresh fruit)

Dinner
　Stuffed broiled salmon
　　5 oz. salmon fillet
　　1 oz. bread stuffing mix
　　1 tablespoon chopped onion
　　1 tablespoon diced celery
　　1 teaspoon canola oil
　1/2 cup rice
　1/2 cup broccoli with 1 teaspoon butter
　1 cup skim milk

Snack
　5 sandwich cookies

(continued)

Menu #2

Breakfast

Hot cereal
- ½ cup cooked oatmeal
- 2 tablespoons raisins
- 1 teaspoon butter

1 cup orange juice

Lunch

Taco salad
- 2 oz. tortilla chips
- 2 oz. ground turkey, sautéed in 2 teaspoons sunflower oil
- ½ cup black beans
- ½ cup lettuce
- 2 slices tomato
- 1 oz. cheddar cheese
- 2 tablespoons salsa
- ½ cup avocado
- 1 teaspoon lime juice

Snack

1 cheese stick, ½ cup fresh fruit

Dinner

Spinach lasagna
- 1 cup lasagna noodles
- ⅓ cup cooked spinach
- ½ cup ricotta cheese
- ½ cup tomato sauce
- 1 oz. mozzarella cheese
- 1 whole wheat dinner roll
- 1 cup skim milk

Snack

- ½ oz. almonds, 2 tablespoons raisins
- ¼ cup fresh fruit

Menu #3

Breakfast

Cold cereal
- 1 cup bran flakes
- 1 cup skim milk
- 1 banana

1 slice wheat bread (with 1 teaspoon butter)

½ cup fruit juice

Lunch

Tuna sandwich
- 2 slices bread
- 3 oz. tuna
- 2 teaspoons mayonnaise
- 1 tablespoon celery
- ¼ cup lettuce
- 2 slices tomato

1 piece fruit

Snack

- 5 crackers
- 2 oz. cheese

Dinner

- 3 oz. roasted chicken breast
- 1 large baked sweet potato
- ½ cup peas and onions (with 1 teaspoon olive oil)
- 1 dinner roll (with 1 teaspoon butter)
- 1 cup salad greens with 3 teaspoons dressing

Snack

1 cup frozen yogurt or ice cream

(continued)

Menu #4

Breakfast
   1 wheat English muffin with 2 teaspoons butter
      and 1 tablespoon jam
   1 medium grapefruit
   1 cup milk

Lunch
   2 cups bean soup (1¼ cup vegetable soup,
      ½ cup beans)
   1 bread stick
   8 baby carrots
   1 oz. cheese

Snack
   1 hard-boiled egg

Dinner
   Rigatoni with meat sauce
      1 cup rigatoni pasta
      ½ cup tomato sauce
      2 oz. lean cooked beef sautéed in 2 teaspoons
         vegetable oil
      3 tablespoons Parmesan cheese
   Spinach salad
      1 cup spinach
      ½ cup tangerine slices
      ½ oz. chopped walnuts
      3 teaspoons oil and vinegar dressing

Snack
   1 cup yogurt

Menu #5

Breakfast
   Cold cereal
      1 cup shredded wheat
      1 tablespoon raisins
      1 cup skim milk
   1 banana
   1 slice wheat toast with 1 teaspoon margarine
      and 1 teaspoon jelly

Lunch
   Turkey sandwich
      2 slices of bread
      ¼ cup lettuce
      2 slices tomato
      3 oz. turkey
      1 tablespoon mayonnaise
      1 teaspoon mustard
   ½ cup apple slices

Snack
   3 mini candy bars

Dinner
   5 oz. grilled steak
   ¾ cup mashed potatoes and 2 teaspoons
      margarine
   ½ cup steamed carrots with 1 tablespoon honey
   1 dinner roll with 1 teaspoon margarine

Snack
   1 cup frozen yogurt or ice cream

(continued)

Menu #6

Breakfast
French toast
   2 slices bread
   1 egg
   2 teaspoons margarine
   2 tablespoons maple syrup
½ medium grapefruit

Lunch
Vegetarian chili on baked potato
   1 cup kidney beans
   ½ cup tomato sauce
   3 tablespoons chopped onion
   1 oz. cheddar cheese
   1 teaspoon vegetable oil
   1 medium baked potato
1 piece fruit or 1 cup fresh fruit

Snack
1 cup yogurt

Dinner
Hawaiian pizza
   2 slices cheese pizza
   1 oz. Canadian bacon
   ¼ cup pineapple
   2 tablespoons mushrooms
   2 tablespoons onion
Green salad with 3 teaspoons dressing
1 cup skim milk

Snack
5 whole wheat crackers
⅛ cup hummus
½ cup fruit

Menu #7

Breakfast
Pancakes
   3 buckwheat pancakes with 2 teaspoons butter
   2 tablespoons maple syrup
½ cup strawberries
1 cup milk

Lunch
Clam chowder
   3 oz. canned clams
   ¾ cup mixed vegetables
   1 cup canned tomatoes
10 wheat crackers
1 piece of fruit
1 oz. piece of cheese

Snack
1 cup yogurt
1 oz. sunflower seeds

Dinner
Vegetable stir fry
   4 oz. tofu
   ¼ cup red and green peppers
   ½ cup bok choy
   2 tablespoons vegetable oil
1 cup rice

Snack
5 cookies

The ACT Skill

The ACT skill means using Adaptive Coping Techniques. When you begin to feel the urge to engage in bulimic behaviors, use the FEEL skill to get an understanding of the feelings that you are having along with urges that trigger your behaviors. Then, follow the steps of the ACT skill to find a way to soothe, distract, or problem-solve without binge eating, purging, or restricting food. The next page includes a list of ideas and suggestions for using the ACT skill. Ideas from your planned activities can be used for adaptive coping. You can also use your skill cards between sessions to help remind you to practice your coping techniques.

At first, the ACT skill might be difficult to use because you may have been using your bulimic behaviors to manage some of your problems or feelings for a long time. We encourage you to practice the ACT skill each day.

Adaptive	• Use the FEEL skill to get ready to ACT. • Can you identify your urge? • Can you identify your need? • Can you manage the urge and meet the need in a healthy way?
Coping	• Is there something you can do to solve the core problem? • Is this a situation that cannot be changed? • Can you change things if you wait? • Is it a time to self-soothe? • Is it a time to distract yourself? • Would your eating disorder behaviors really help?
Technique	• Coping is a skill that can be learned. • Coping efforts improve with practice. • What might help you to cope more effectively right now? • How can you meet your need differently?

Examples of Three Ways to Use the Act Skill

Self-Soothe	Self-Distract	Act to Change the Problem
• Take a bath • Listen to music • Take a walk • Drink herbal tea • Be with your pet • Look at soothing images	• Call or text a friend • Use the computer • Read a book • Exercise • Play the piano • Do some type of craft or project	• Avoid a restaurant that triggers bulimic behavior • End a problematic relationship • Tell someone why you are upset • Plan to see friends to avoid being alone during the weekend • Make a decision to join a singing group or choir to do something that you enjoy

The GOAL Skill

The GOAL skill is included in your treatment because setting small, adaptive, and attainable goals is important to your recovery, as well as to life in general. The GOAL skill encourages you to set short-term goals in areas that you are trying to change. This could include efforts to increase the number of meals you eat or the number of times you practice skills per day, adopting a different interpersonal style with certain people in your life, or trying to modify the way you treat yourself.

Below is a description of the GOAL skill. It starts out by asking how you want to change over the next 5 years. That time may seem far away, but changes in the next 5 years will be based on decisions that are made in the next days and weeks. Consequently, you will see throughout the GOAL skill that we are focused on setting goals for short periods of time. Good luck as you set goals for your treatment and your life.

Goals	• In 5 years, what do you hope will be true about your life? • Is the eating disorder part of your plan for the next 5 years? • What parts of your life do you want to develop or change in the next 5 years? • If you don't have goals, what interferes with setting some?
Objectives	• What goal are you working on today? • What will help you right now to reach your goal? • What could set you back in reaching your goal?
Affect	• If you reach your objective for today, how will you feel? What will it mean to you? • How can you manage urges today that could interfere with your objective?
Life-moments	• In this treatment we encourage you to try and change each moment. • This means trying to make choices and manage each situation you encounter without eating disorder behavior.

It is important to understand that when you set goals there will always be things in life that interfere with the attainment of your goals. You can be feeling particularly badly, you may be sick, unexpected and difficult events may occur, or you may just not have enough time. During your treatment, you and your clinician will be trying to understand what interferes with reaching your goals as well as how you can effectively attain them.

It is also important to check in with yourself about how you feel when setting particular goals. Your goals should be authentic in nature and truly valued by you. Of course, there may be some goals that you truly value but may have mixed feelings, including fear, about trying to achieve. These types of goals may include some of your eating disorder behaviors including binge eating, purging, and food restriction. If you are ambivalent or confused about setting certain goals, it is important to talk about it with your clinician to gain clarity and understanding.

Choosing a Focus for Your Treatment

You have completed an important phase of your treatment, and it is important to decide with your therapist what direction you should take next. It is recommended that you work with your therapist to identify those aspects of your daily life that might be most associated with your bulimic behavior and, if changed, would help you to feel more satisfied and make more adaptive choices.

Here are some possibilities for this next treatment phase:

1. **Working on food and emotions.** You may still have difficulty eating regular, planned meals and snacks as well as tolerating the emotions associated with your eating patterns or changes in your eating patterns. If so, your therapist may recommend continuing to closely monitor your food consumption while working on adaptive coping with the emotions that arise. It is important to continue to work on the CARE, FEEL, and ACT skills and attempt to reduce binge eating to avoid or escape painful emotions or problems.

2. **Relationships.** Many people who have bulimia nervosa have difficulties with interpersonal relationships. If you have concerns about the way you relate to others, relationships might be an important target for this phase of your treatment. People with eating disorders often struggle with being too submissive, blaming others, acting too shy or withdrawn, or feeling unable to express themselves effectively. If you have these concerns, you may want to consider focusing on relationship patterns.

3. **The way I treat myself.** Many individuals who have bulimic episodes struggle with the way they treat themselves. They may be very rigid and self-controlling, self-critical, or treat themselves recklessly and then regret the consequences. If you recognize the way you treat yourself as something that concerns you, you may wish to consider this focus during the next phase.

4. **Not living up to my standards.** Many people who have bulimia nervosa strive for unrealistic goals that are exceedingly difficult to achieve and then feel inadequate when they believe that they have failed to meet their standards. If you find that you often feel inadequate or like you have failed, you may wish to consider this particular target in the next phase of your treatment.

It is also possible that several of these issues affect you, and you may wish to address several of them in this next phase of treatment. You and your therapist can work together to decide what will be most helpful to you.

Beginning to Make SEA Changes

One way to think about your eating disorder is in terms of **situations, emotions, and actions.** Situations are those experiences or environmental cues that can affect us emotionally and behaviorally, like having an argument or failing an exam. They might be something simple like eating a meal or noticing that your pants fit you differently than before.

Situations like these lead to emotions. For example, you might feel sadness when a relationship ends or feel anxious sitting in the doctor's office. These are both examples of situations associated with particular feelings. Hopefully, you are beginning to get a clearer sense of your typical emotional responses to specific situations.

When situations occur that cause certain feelings, how do you act? Consider Jane. She has recently been working hard on a project at her office and just received criticism from her manager about her performance on this project. She felt angry, frustrated, and sad. She left work early, stopped to buy food, drove home, and binge-ate all afternoon and evening. Here, the *situation* (criticism from manager) led to *emotions* (angry, frustrated, sad), which triggered *actions* (isolation, binge eating).

The combination of situations (S), emotions (E), and actions (A) is what we call a SEA unit. The goal of treatment is to promote change in the SEA unit, or what we like to call "SEA Change." SEA Change is important in recovery. In order to stop bulimic behavior, it is essential to become aware of situations that are a problem for you and the emotions that they cause. Ultimately, you may learn to take different actions in the face of particular emotions and manage situations more effectively so negative emotions are decreased. Working on your homework and seeing your therapist are important parts of treatment, but any changes to help you stop bulimic behavior have to be practiced in real-life situations. For example, if tomorrow at 2 o'clock in the afternoon you experience a stressful situation, you are feeling upset, and you are struggling with urges to binge-eat or purge, it will be in that moment that you need to practice coping with the emotions using healthy strategies rather than bulimic behavior.

Handout 7.3 is a blank SEA Change Diary and Handout 7.4 is a sample completed SEA Change Diary that illustrates how you will use this form. We know that you have been keeping track of what you have been eating, but this diary is different and can be used along with your CARE forms. Please write down times when you have binge-eating and/or purging episodes or urges to binge-eat. Write down bulimic behavior or urges in the *Action* column. Think about the emotions that you had along with these behaviors or urges. What did you experience immediately beforehand? Write down those feelings in the *Emotion* column. Then, think about the situation that may have triggered the emotions and write this down in the *Situation* column. Finally, ask yourself what *function* you think the bulimic behavior may have served. This process will help you to become aware of important situations as they occur in your daily experience, the emotions they cause, and the actions you choose to help you deal with these emotions. As you learn about your patterns using the SEA Change Diary, you will learn to use more effective actions to cope instead of eating disorder behavior. We encourage you to bring your SEA Change Diaries to all of your therapy sessions with as many SEA examples as you can identify each week.

SEA Change Diary

When using the blank SEA Change Diary, please list any instances in which you had a bulimic episode or urges to binge and/or purge in the **Action** column. List the **Situation** that occurred before the binge or urge to binge as well as any **Emotions** that were associated with the situation. Also, attempt to describe what you think you needed in that situation and your hopes about how the bulimic episode would help you.

Situation	Emotion	Action

What I needed in the situation/the function of the binge:

Situation	Emotion	Action

What I needed in the situation/the function of the binge:

Sample Completed SEA Change Diary

Situation	Emotion	Action
Had a fight on the phone with my sister after she canceled our plans	Sad Lonely Hurt Frustrated Abandoned	Bingeing instead of sticking with planned snack

What I needed in the situation/the function of the binge:

I wanted a break from my life.

Situation	Emotion	Action
Didn't get enough sleep last night, stayed up to watch TV	Bored Tired Guilty for almost falling asleep	Ate more than planned on during staff meeting then vomited after the meeting

What I needed in the situation/the function of the binge:

Give myself something to do, keep me engaged in the meeting.

Beginning to Address My Relationship with Myself and Others

So far, your treatment has focused on helping you to develop healthy eating patterns and better coping strategies. Hopefully, you have also begun to identify your feelings more clearly. It will be important to continue to pay careful attention to those feelings and to develop skills to help you effectively manage your feelings.

In this phase of your treatment, the focus will shift to relationships and also the way that you view and treat yourself. The way we relate to others and ourselves can have a significant impact on how we feel, as well as how we behave. Often, bulimic behaviors help us to deal with negative feelings. Therefore, we believe that if you change your relationship patterns with yourself and others, your bulimic behavior will also improve.

As your treatment moves forward, we **strongly encourage you to continue working on your FEEL, CARE, ACT, and GOAL skills.** Working on problems in relationships or your views of yourself without continuing to address your eating patterns, feelings, and coping skills is unlikely to be as effective as focusing on all of these areas of your life. We will continue to work with you on monitoring your eating behavior, even as we begin to focus more on relationships and other factors that may play a role in your eating patterns. Hopefully, this process will also help you to see how your bulimic behavior relates to specific issues in your life. Therefore, it will be **important for you to continue using your meal plans and daily food records** and to bring them to each of your sessions. In particular, pay careful attention to the last column of your food records so that you can make notes about personal and emotional factors that are related to your eating patterns.

Possible Things to Change: My Relationships to Other People

It is possible that your bulimic behavior is in some way related to your interpersonal relationships and emotions. Various interpersonal relationships can cause significant emotional problems. Consider your typical way of relating to important people in your life. We call these your interpersonal patterns. Some people seem to get along well with everybody, but in truth most people struggle with relationships in some way. Some people have difficulty with a certain kind of person. Other people have difficulty with just about everybody. Some people have difficulty with one person, and one person only. It is important to wonder what might be contributing to your difficult relationships. If you struggle with one relationship, what is it about that relationship that makes it a problem? Does the person say or do things that often upset you? Do you not know how to respond when the person puts you in a difficult situation? Are you constantly trying to please or satisfy the person? Are you trying to get away from the person and they are not letting it happen? It will be important to really think about the particular circumstances that contribute to the difficulties you are having in your relationships.

You might have an overall strategy in relationships that is not working well for you; if you notice you are having problems in several relationships over time, this may be the case. Maybe you try too hard to make people happy. Maybe you expect too much from people. Maybe you give too much to people and they take advantage of you. Maybe you are afraid to enter relationships and consequently don't give much to other people because of fear. Maybe you blame other people for some of the problems you are facing. Whatever the issue is, it is important to think about it and talk about it with your therapist. See if you can find ways to improve your relationships in some small way. Doing so could significantly help your recovery as it might help you feel better about yourself and reduce your negative emotions.

Below, we will outline two different kinds of situations. The first has to do with difficulty in one particular relationship. The second has to do struggles with a series of relationships. See which situation fits you best and think about ways you might be able to make some changes.

"I Am Fine with Just about Everybody Except One Person"

Some people get along quite well with a variety of people but struggle with one particular relationship. It might be a particularly important relationship, such as a spouse, significant other, parent, child, or a particularly close friend. This relationship may serve as a trigger for your binge eating, and it will be important to try to identify what it is about this relationship that makes it so difficult. Are there differences in power (like a parent–child relationship)? Does this person repeatedly fail to meet your needs, but you stay with him or her? Do you have difficulty expressing your needs and wishes to this person? Are there clear examples in which this person has mistreated you? Is there a history of this person violating your trust?

Regardless of the specific nature of the problem in this particular relationship, it may be important to your recovery to try to make changes. We generally recommend that you attempt to approach the person and address your differences in the hope that it will increase satisfaction in the relationship. If such change does not then happen, we generally suggest trying to reduce contact with the person or change the degree of closeness in the relationship.

(continued)

The following steps might be useful to try:

1. Approach the other person in an effort to express the frustrations, disappointments, problematic interactions, or other aspects of the relationship that pose problems. Express yourself clearly and respectfully using the SAID skill (see Handout 7.7). Try to let the person know precisely what the problem is (from your perspective) and what you would like to see different.

2. Monitor the relationship for change. Recognize that change sometimes comes slowly. Assume that you will need to continue to address problems if things are to improve. Asserting yourself once is unlikely to be sufficient to make lasting change. You will probably need to use the SAID skill repeatedly to change the relationship.

3. Carefully decide whether change has occurred and, if so, whether you are satisfied.

4. If you decide that further change is unlikely, how can you modify the nature of this relationship to reduce your exposure to its problem aspects? Can you minimize contact? Can you limit the relationship so that its problematic aspects are removed? Can you and the other person come to an agreement that some degree of disengagement may be a beneficial solution?

5. If the relationship does not change and continues to be a significant source of emotional distress and a trigger for bulimic behavior, you may need to consider separating from or ending this relationship.

Make sure you talk about this relationship in your therapy and keep an eye out for how it affects your eating in your SEA Change Diaries.

"None of My Relationships Work! Why Does This Happen?"

If you notice that most of your relationships have been problematic, disappointing, and difficult, it might be important to ask yourself the following questions. Is it possible that you have learned some behavior patterns or expectations about relationships that do not work well for you? Could you be too shy, too dramatic, or too aggressive? Everyone has particular styles of relating. Such styles are products of our genetics and our collection of life experiences. Healthy interpersonal functioning involves finding relationships that fit well with your patterns *and* allow you to be comfortable in relationships. Sometimes you might have to tolerate others' relationship styles and work with the other person to find cooperative solutions or ways to relate.

If you notice that you have had problems in several relationships, you might want to consider changing the patterns you use in these relationships. In the next section, we identify some key patterns and ways to change these patterns.

Identifying Interpersonal Patterns

Ideally, our interpersonal behavior reflects our *conscious* choice about how to behave in a particular situation at a given moment in time. However, often our interpersonal choices reflect *automatic or habitual* patterns of relating to other people that we have developed over time and we simply keep repeating. Sometimes these interpersonal patterns are ways for us to try to cope with negative feelings about ourselves or our feelings of not being "good enough." If you think that others are likely to reject you because you think you are inadequate, you are likely to feel bad. In your efforts to avoid rejection, you may make relationship choices that result in more emotional pain and make bulimic behavior worse.

In ICAT, it is important for you to gain a clear understanding of your own interpersonal patterns, as well as the patterns of those around you. Below are descriptions of some common relationship patterns. See if you can begin to identify your typical pattern.

(continued)

Patterns That People with Eating Disorders Often Report

The following patterns, described by Dr. Lorna Benjamin (1996), can increase negative emotions. Do you engage in any of them on a regular basis?

1. **Submit to others.** Some people behave submissively, hoping that others will tell them what to do. Others behave submissively out of fear that if they don't, they might be punished or rejected. Submissive patterns are characterized by giving up your own thoughts or intentions and simply "going along with things." Many people who tend to submit also report hidden feelings of anger and hostility, which they fail to express, or express indirectly.

2. **Walling off from others.** Some people tend to angrily pull away from others. It is as though they are saying, "I don't have any interest in being close to you." They may feel that if they try to discuss the situation, they will be hurt further and consequently things will only worsen.

3. **Blaming.** This pattern refers to hostile, often reckless efforts to harm, criticize, and belittle another person. The goal is to get him or her to act in some way you want.

4. **Expecting more than others want to offer.** Some people assume that others want the same thing they want. This is often not true and may result in others pulling away because they feel manipulated or not respected.

Finally, we would like to point out two alternative patterns that may help in your recovery as described below:

1. **Express or assert with others.** Clearly, honestly, and openly express your opinions. Simply state what is on your mind—what you think, how you feel, or what you would like to see happen. "Lay your cards on the table" so that others know where you stand.

The second pattern is about the way you could treat others. It may also reflect how you wish to be treated. If so, look for this pattern in others when establishing new relationships.

2. **Affirm and accept.** Accept others in a friendly way, even if they differ from you. Don't try to change others' opinions or perspectives.

These last two patterns do not guarantee happiness in relationships, but they are reasonable approaches to getting along with others. It is important for each of us to be able to express our opinions freely, but we must also accept the consequences of our opinions. Not everybody is going to like what we say. It can be a significant problem if you are in relationships in which you are not at least somewhat accepted, and are expected to change or submit to others' wishes. At the same time, it is unwise to think that important people in our lives will accept everything we do. In general, the people we rely on most should be people who basically accept us, and when we differ, both parties state their opinion, tolerate the difference, and accept that as part of the relationship.

The SAID Skill

The SAID skill is designed to help you deal with relationships more effectively. It is a set of reminders for carefully and sensitively expressing your thoughts and desires to other people. Although others may not always appreciate what you think or want, it may be important for you to express these ideas. However, sometimes expressing yourself can pose problems in a relationship. Consider these risks carefully before you decide to assert yourself. Try to distinguish asserting yourself from aggressively attacking somebody with your words or body language. Remember to express your thoughts or feelings as honestly as possible in a respectful manner. If you find yourself criticizing or blaming other people, you are probably no longer asserting yourself respectfully.

Sensitively	• Use the FEEL skill before you speak (SAID). • Dealing with relationship problems may be difficult, but it is part of your recovery. • Express your ideas, feelings, and needs respectfully. • Others might not change in response to your requests, but communicating with them is still valuable.
Assert	• You may want to "lay your cards on the table" honestly. • You may want to express an emotion, either positive or negative. • You may want to ask for something.
Ideas	• What is your opinion? • What do you believe? • What do you want? • What do you need?
Desires	• You may want to ask someone to do something for you. • You may want to express a desire to be closer to someone. • You may want to express a desire to separate from someone. • You may want to ask someone to do more or less of something.

The Development of Interpersonal Patterns

Interpersonal patterns refer to the way each of us tends to relate to other people. Even though we may differ in our interpersonal behavior when we are with different people or in different situations, we each have a general pattern of behavior with others that is fairly stable. It can be difficult to determine how our interpersonal patterns developed. There is evidence to suggest that our genetic heritage determines something about our typical interpersonal patterns. There is also good reason to believe that experience, or an accumulation of experiences, can significantly influence our patterns. Most often, it is not a single experience that shapes our patterns, but the day-in and day-out experiences that we have with particular other people.

Below, we would like you to think about the origins of your interpersonal patterns. This is not an exercise about identifying a particular person who you can blame for any problems you are experiencing. Rather, the goal of this exercise is to understand what may have contributed to the development of your current patterns. In understanding the origin of your patterns, you can more carefully evaluate them and determine if you wish to continue them.

The answers to these questions are not likely to be simple. You may have to think about them quite a bit before you can put together some answers.

1. Based on what you have learned so far, what are your key interpersonal patterns (e.g., submissive, withdrawn, aggressive)?

   _____

   _____

   _____

2. When are you most likely to see these patterns?

   _____

   _____

   _____

3. Below, rate how much each item influenced your development of these patterns.

   _____

   _____

   A. Early relationships (e.g., parents, siblings, peers)? If yes, please describe:

   _____

   _____

   B. School? If yes, please describe.

   _____

   _____

(continued)

C. Work? If yes, please describe:

_____

_____

D. Marriage or dating relationships? Your parents' relationship to one another? If yes, please describe:

_____

_____

4. Do you see any negative consequences of continuing to engage in your pattern?

_____

_____

_____

5. Do you have any desire to modify your pattern? Why?

_____

_____

_____

A. If not, what do you expect would happen if you did try to change?

_____

_____

B. What could interfere with learning or trying new patterns?

_____

_____

Tips on Modifying Interpersonal Patterns

As you become more aware of your interpersonal patterns, you may decide that you would like to change the way you behave in specific relationships. This is entirely possible and will require you to do the following things:

1. Continue to pay careful attention to your patterns in current close relationships.

2. Think about specific ways in which you would like to change these patterns.

3. Role-play in your mind specific things you would like to say or do in relationships and rehearse this new pattern repeatedly.

4. To improve your chances for successful change, plan the changes you are going to make first. Do not impulsively decide to try to do something different in the middle of a situation.

5. After you have tried out new patterns, evaluate them. Think about what went well and what you would like to do differently next time.

6. In intimate relationships, explain to the other individual why it is important for you to make these changes. This helps others to understand the nature of the change that they are seeing.

7. Be prepared for the possibility that some people will not like your change. If you continue to believe that it is right for you, continue to develop the pattern.

8. Praise and reward yourself for trying to make change, even if it does not work out perfectly.

9. Sometimes journaling or writing letters can be helpful in clarifying and expressing your thoughts and feelings about a relationship, as well as what you would like to change. After you have written the letter, you can decide whether or not to send it.

10. Remind yourself that the goal is not for you to blame and change other people: it is to change your own patterns.

Dealing with Specific Patterns

Depending on the particular pattern you are trying to change, there are some specific changes you may want to consider.

Submit Pattern

If you have been engaging in a submit pattern, consider the following suggestions:

1. Clearly identify what it feels like when others are controlling you or when you are repeatedly submitting.

2. When you are in a situation, attempt to identify what feelings **you** are experiencing at the moment.

3. Try and find situations in which you can state your opinion or your feelings about a situation. Do this gradually.

(continued)

4. If you are attempting to overcome a submit pattern in an intimate relationship, let the other person know that you need to make this change. This will help him or her prepare for the changes you are about to make.

5. Don't expect people to like the changes you are making. Some people like others who are passive and submissive. However, this does not mean you should remain submissive.

6. Develop your assertive behavior using the SAID skill. Assertive expression involves clearly and simply expressing your thoughts and feelings without requiring the other person to behave in a particular manner. The goal is to identify your thoughts, feelings, and wishes at a given time and then choose whether or not it is important for you to express them. If it is, proceed to express yourself. Be respectful of others in how you express yourself.

7. Learning to be assertive after a long period of submission can be scary. Recognize that you might feel tense when you are beginning to increase your assertive behavior. You may find that you cry. This is to be expected and reflects the fact that you are doing something new and having new feelings. That is progress. Use your FEEL skill as you practice being assertive.

8. Do not expect other people to stop being controlling or dominating simply because you were assertive once or twice. In the beginning, others in your life may become more controlling in an attempt to get you to return to your old submissive pattern. You will need to repeatedly practice assertive behaviors so the new pattern can develop and others can adjust.

Wall-Off Pattern (Withdrawal)

If you tend to avoid getting close to people (perhaps out of fear or frustration) or disengage because you are angry or scared, consider the following suggestions:

1. Try to identify one or two relationships where you can practice being "closer" to those people. Pick reasonably safe relationships.

2. Focus on trying to open up to these people, perhaps sharing feelings, opinions, or ideas. You are likely to get a better response if you can express yourself in a warm way that recognizes the other person's position, for example, "I really appreciate those times when you have asked me how my day was even when I know you had a really hard day yourself."

3. Look for opportunities to spend more time with these individuals.

4. Be careful not to go overboard. Don't overwhelm people you have been avoiding by making too many demands on them or expressing too many opinions or feelings at first. Start out small and see how they respond. Think about how you expressed your thoughts and feelings (e.g., your tone of voice, what you said, and your facial expression).

5. If you are trying to overcome a withdrawal pattern with someone you were once very close with (e.g., family member, close friend, spouse), focus on sharing your feelings. Consider whether or not you need to talk about what happened previously in the relationship that increased the distance. Consider whether or not you might benefit from constructively acknowledging any anger and let the other person know how you have been feeling.

(continued)

6. Try to do nice things for other people. Compliment them, do favors for them, give appropriate indications of your friendship (e.g., cards or small gifts). Put yourself in their shoes and imagine what they might appreciate. Think of these acts as gifts you give to another without any expectation of what you will get in return.

7. Keep experimenting with increasing your trust of others. Allow others to do things for you and practice graciously accepting their kindness.

Unrealistic Expectations of Others

If you have reason to believe that you may expect too much of others or expect them to act in a particular way, which causes problems, consider the following suggestions:

1. Have people suggested to you, directly or indirectly, that you ask too much of them or that you tend to believe that other people should do things for you?

2. What is your personal understanding of how others should relate to you? Do you feel like you expect others to help you manage your life?

3. Do you ever talk to important people in your life about this issue? Have you discussed with them whether or not you expect too much of them?

4. Do you work on trying to be independent? Is that difficult for you?

5. Do you sometimes feel like people should be willing to help you or others just don't understand what you are going through? If that is true, do you think that has a negative impact on your relationships with others?

6. When people do help you and provide assistance, do you have a real sense of appreciation for their effort?

7. How do you feel about helping other people out? Do you believe that there is a real give-and-take in your relationships? Do you feel you are working together with the other person?

8. If you are not sure whether or not you may be expecting too much of others, think about asking some of your closest friends or family.

Blame Pattern

If you frequently engage in a blaming pattern (you might not be sure you do, but others may think you do), consider the following suggestions:

1. Do you find yourself frequently getting angry at people or blaming them for your problems? Have others suggested you are too aggressive or angry?

2. Identify why you are blaming or attacking. What do you hope this will accomplish? Are you trying to get control or distance in relationship to certain people? Consider the short-term versus long-term costs of blaming and attacking others.

3. If you are trying to get someone to admit they are wrong or conform to your wishes, then blaming or attacking might not be the most useful approach. Frequently, it results in more fighting or in the other person withdrawing.

(continued)

4. If you truly want others to understand what you are experiencing or what you want, consider *assertive behavior* (see the **SAID skill**). Identify your thoughts, feelings, or wishes and make a decision as to whether or not you wish to express them to the person in a respectful manner.

5. Be prepared for the possibility that you may not get what you want. Practice acceptance. Simply because we want things does not mean that we always get them. Not getting what you want *right now* does not mean you will *never* get what you want.

6. Avoid automatically resorting to anger, criticism, and hostility when people disappoint you.

7. If you notice that you are feeling extremely angry in an interpersonal situation, take a break and calm down before you attempt to be assertive with the other person. It is hard to be effectively assertive when you are experiencing the physical effects of anger.

8. If you are using your anger to try to get some distance or space from people, consider simple separation rather than hostility. That is, find a way to get the space you need without resorting to anger. You may want to let the other person know that you need to take a break but are willing to discuss the situation again later.

9. If you are using your anger to try to control another person's behavior, try using assertive expression to let them know what you want. However, be prepared if they don't do exactly what you want.

People with bulimic behaviors often struggle with these patterns. As you can see, assertive behavior becomes important in changing all of these patterns. We believe it is important to identify your true feelings and thoughts and then decide whether or not you wish to express them. This decision should be based on what will lead to your desired outcome and not just on what is comfortable in the moment. The ability to effectively and respectfully express your feelings and sentiments to other people is an important skill.

The REAL Skill

It is common for individuals with bulimic behaviors to feel dissatisfied and not good enough. The first step in changing these negative attitudes is to identify how you actually see yourself. For example, note the aspects of yourself that you like and some you do not like. You also need to become aware of the standards you are setting for yourself. What do you expect from yourself? Frequently, individuals with bulimic behaviors have extremely high standards for themselves, which are difficult to attain. This can lead to a very negative view of the self. As part of treatment we need to help you develop a realistic picture of yourself as well as keeping your expectations flexible and realistic.

The REAL skill asks you to monitor your self-standards in the moment and figure out whether or not those standards are reasonable and fair. We also encourage you to take a closer look at the positive aspects about yourself that you may be overlooking or downplaying.

Realistic	• Use the FEEL skill to get ready to be REAL. • Being realistic about yourself means being fair and reasonable. • Draw conclusions based on the present moment, not the past.
Expectations	• Pay attention to the standards you set for yourself. • Are your goals fair and attainable? • If you don't reach a goal, can you credit yourself for trying? • Do the expectations you have for yourself reflect your values or somebody else's?
Affect	• Unrealistic self-standards and self-judgments can make you depressed, anxious, and frustrated. • What would it be like right now to be acceptable or good enough?
Living	• The way you evaluate yourself may affect your life goals. • The way you evaluate yourself may affect relationships. • Are you living your life with goals that you value?

Possible Things to Change: Expectations for Myself

We believe that when your perception of yourself differs from the way that you would ideally like to be, your risk of developing eating problems increases. People who have bulimic behavior often evaluate themselves quite harshly. They tend to believe that they are not good enough.

We would like you to spend some time thinking about how you evaluate yourself. Do you see yourself accurately and completely? Do you hold standards for yourself that are reasonable and attainable, or are they unfair and even unattainable? Would you expect your best friend to live up to your expectations? What will happen to you if you don't begin to change the way you evaluate yourself?

How you evaluate yourself can strongly influence your feelings. Self-evaluation has two components:

1. The way you see your actual self: the characteristics that you believe you possess; how you see yourself as a person.

2. The way you see your desired self: the characteristics that you would like to possess or feel you must possess; how you want to be as a person.

Your desired self is a standard or goal that you compare to your actual self. If the desired and actual self are close to the same, you usually experience a sense of satisfaction and self-acceptance.

However, if your desired self is different from your actual self, you may experience feelings of disappointment, anxiety, and depression. This difference between the actual self as compared to the desired self is referred to as self-discrepancy. It results in feeling inadequate, not good enough. It may also motivate you to try to change yourself so that you can try to live up to your standards.

You may also have difficulty with self-acceptance. Many people who struggle with bulimic behavior strive to become a person very different from whom they naturally are. Are there parts of yourself that you can comfortably accept, and may even make you feel proud or satisfied? Are there parts of yourself that you have particular difficulty accepting? What are they and why do you think it is so difficult to accept them? We recognize that giving up on a dream of being different or of reaching some goal can be hard and emotionally painful. As you work toward self-acceptance, we encourage you to struggle with your emotional reactions in a manner that allows you to come to terms with who you actually are.

Please take a minute to think about some aspect of yourself that you feel is not up to your standard. It could be related to your performance in school or at work, your appearance, your weight, your shape, or a relationship with someone else. When you hold that in your mind, how do you feel? Let the feelings come to you and sit with them as best you can. When you are experiencing these feelings, do you have any urges to try to change something about yourself? After you have finished, write down what you noticed and make sure to discuss it with your therapist.

Notes:

_____

_____

This experience is exactly the kind of thought and feeling process we want to talk about in your therapy. When you are feeling that you are not living up to a standard, remember to ask how it makes you feel and what you want to do about it. This series of steps is the basic idea in the REAL skill. Make sure to tell your therapist about the results of this exercise.

What Do I Wish to Be?

As part of your recovery, we encourage you to think about your goals and the standards you use to judge your accomplishments. All too often, people who have bulimic behavior spend a lot of time thinking about what kind of person they should be or have to be, including their appearance.

As you are thinking about your goals, it might be helpful to wonder what kind of person you would really like to be. This requires you to really think about your personal ideals and wishes. This may or may not include what you or others think you should be or have to be.

Ask yourself the following (and feel free to write notes about what you learn):

1. What kind of person am I without trying to change anything? Are there aspects of my actual self that I am proud of or pleased about?

2. When I feel that I have to be a certain way, where is that "command" coming from? Is it fair and good for me? How does it lead me to treat myself?

3. What do I really want to strive to be as a person? Is this standard for myself fair and reasonable given who I actually am?

Checking My Personal Standards

This exercise is designed to help you become more aware of your standards. List the things you would like to be in the left column. This is your desired self. Then answer each question in the remaining columns. What do you think about your standards?

Description of a part of my desired self (e.g., smart, social, pretty, fit)	Do I meet this standard?	Is my standard fair and reasonable? Is it good for me?

The SPA Skill

The way you treat yourself is very important to your recovery. Many individuals with eating problems struggle with being too self-controlling, self-critical, or self-neglectful. They have difficulty accepting themselves. These types of self-directed behaviors may induce feelings of frustration, hopelessness, and anger. We encourage you to work on efforts to accept yourself and protect yourself both physically and psychologically, especially when you are in treatment and trying to recover. This is not a time to put yourself in risky or problematic situations that threaten your recovery. The SPA skill is a strategy to help you to engage in these self-accepting and self-protecting patterns more consistently.

Self	• Use the FEEL skill to prepare for using the SPA skill. • Think about how you are relating to yourself. • Is the way that you are treating yourself in this moment healthy and adaptive?
Protect	• Recovery means protecting and caring for yourself. • Are you taking care of your needs, including food and eating? • How can you commit to your treatment and recovery as a way of caring for and protecting yourself?
Accept	• Are your goals fair and helpful? • What are you trying to accomplish? • How can you accept yourself and still strive for improvement? • How can you tolerate your limits or personal flaws? • Are there good things about yourself that you are currently ignoring?

Possible Things to Change: The Way I Treat Myself

An important factor to think about in your recovery is the way that you treat yourself. Treating yourself in a hostile or controlling manner can make you feel worse emotionally. Perhaps you criticize yourself or try and control yourself as a way to help you improve as a person, but these actions can make things worse. For example, if you fail to achieve a particular goal you may be really tough on yourself or push yourself to succeed next time. You may view this as a "path to excellence," but it can also cause problems. A different approach is to pursue self-acceptance, which means accepting yourself the way you are, including various flaws and limitations, as well as recognizing your strengths and talents. Self-acceptance may be challenging, but a lack of self-acceptance will lead you to feel chronically frustrated and unhappy as well as putting you at risk of trying to change yourself through unhealthy means. Begin to think about the ways you treat yourself and how that may affect your eating behavior.

Identifying My Patterns of Relationship with Myself

Different people treat themselves very differently, particularly when pursuing a goal. We would like you to begin to think about how you treat yourself. We call this your self-directed behavior. Here are some examples of these behaviors that were described by Dr. Lorna Benjamin (1996).

1. **Self-acceptance.** This pattern involves accepting oneself and appearance with a realistic awareness of shortcomings as well as strengths. It refers to those times in which a person can comfortably be "as is."

2. **Self-protection.** This style is a way of warmly looking after one's own best interests. This pattern differs from self-control (below) in that one gently and lovingly protects oneself rather than tightly controlling the self.

3. **Self-control.** This is a pattern of tightly controlling oneself in an effort to do things right.

4. **Self-criticism.** This pattern is a tendency to attack or criticize the self without much thought about the consequences of the behavior. This pattern of self-directed hostility may include self-punishment.

5. **Self-neglect.** This is a pattern of reckless neglect of the self, letting oneself go without care or concern about the outcome. Putting the self in risky or unhealthy situations is an example of self-neglect.

Which of these patterns are familiar to you?

_____

_____

_____

_____

_____

_____

_____

_____

Tips on Changing the Way You Treat Yourself

We believe it is important to develop new and friendlier ways of treating yourself. The goal is to balance accepting yourself as you are with demanding that you change. If you simply accept yourself as you are, you limit your ability to grow and develop. If you only demand changes of yourself, you will be chronically dissatisfied and unhappy with yourself. Below are the more common patterns of people with bulimia and suggestions for how to change them.

Excessive Self-Control

People who display this pattern are frequently worried that they have not done enough or performed well enough. Because they often worry that others will find them unacceptable in some way, they try to maintain unreasonably high standards to make sure that they are acceptable to others. If you struggle with this pattern, here are some suggestions:

1. Challenge the idea that perfection is attainable or that it is necessary for happiness and contentment.
2. Seriously consider your desired self (who and how you want to be). Is it realistic? Have you ever attained it? What do you imagine will happen to you if you ever do attain it? Can you see yourself as "good enough?"
3. Identify goals and standards that cause you to stretch your abilities but are sensitive to who you actually are. Make sure *you* want to pursue these standards.
4. Give yourself breaks, relax, and make the time to take care of yourself. Even elite athletes realize that success comes from a balance of hard work and recovery. Work on self-protection by gently looking after your best interests.
5. Consider spontaneity. Pay attention to the first thought that comes to your mind or allow yourself to consider spontaneous actions that are not necessarily productive.
6. Develop and enjoy humor, both within yourself and humor that you share with others.
7. Forgive yourself for not attaining your goals.
8. Consider how your eating patterns might reflect too much self-control.

Self-Neglect

If you engage in a pattern of frequently letting yourself go, drifting without much direction, or following your interests or pursuits without much thought of the consequences, consider the following ideas:

1. Challenge the idea that you can always impulsively do whatever it is you want to do when you want to do it.
2. Examine whether you are afraid of progress, failing, or taking responsibility in your life.
3. Begin to develop a plan for yourself. Identify basic goals regarding things such as school, work, or other activities that interest you.

(continued)

4. Develop a plan of action. Be flexible and willing to change if the plan doesn't work.

5. Reward yourself for accomplishing goals, no matter how small they are.

6. Develop an attitude that it is important to take care of yourself. Ask yourself before doing something, "Is this good self-care?"; "Am I being self-protective?"; "Is this the way I would treat a cherished loved one?" If the answer is no to any of these questions, reconsider your actions.

7. Make sleep and activity a priority for yourself. Adequate sleep is an essential part of self-care and will also help with your eating patterns. Moving your bedtime earlier by even as little as 30 minutes can make a difference in how you feel. Activity can take many forms including regular exercise, but the most important part of activity is that it is healthy and adaptive. Consider ways that you can increase your activity level in the form of travel, walking, hobbies, and exercise.

8. Consider how your eating patterns might reflect self-neglect. Review the CARE skill and focus on changing your eating behaviors as part of your self-care.

Self-Blame

If you find that you are often self-critical or feel inadequate, unacceptable, or unlovable, consider the following suggestions:

1. Recognize that no one is perfect and that everyone makes mistakes and has shortcomings. Strive for excellence, not perfection.

2. Continue to work on identifying when and where you first developed your belief that you are undeserving, unlovable, or inadequate.

3. Continue to challenge the accuracy of the belief that you are inadequate or undeserving. In what ways are you adequate and deserving?

4. Emphasize the acceptable aspects of yourself, no matter how small you think they are.

5. Be fair. Would you treat a close friend or child the way that you are treating yourself?

6. Work on forgiving yourself for your perceived shortcomings or inadequacies.

7. When you do make a mistake, identify your role in it, make apologies if necessary, and try to move on.

8. Consider how your eating patterns might be a way of blaming yourself.

The ideal pattern of relating to yourself includes self-acceptance, tolerance of mistakes, motivation to improve yourself, and plans that will help you to accomplish reasonable goals based on realistic standards.

The Wait Skill

Remaining Aware of High-Risk Situations Following Treatment

Most often, people who complete treatment have made significant changes and will continue to do so even after this treatment ends. As you continue to practice your skills and incorporate them into your life, you will be more effective at coping with situations and emotions without relying on binge eating to avoid or escape difficult feelings. However, there may be times after treatment ends when your urges to binge-eat increase. Struggling with urges to binge-eat is normal and an anticipated part of your recovery.

In this final phase of your treatment, we will discuss ways of preventing relapse. The skill for this is the WAIT skill. It emphasizes the importance of monitoring your impulses (or urges) each day. As the WAIT skill emphasizes, recovery is more likely if you remain aware of yourself, the situations you encounter, and your emotions in those situations. Initially, you may have strong urges to return to your old eating patterns, but with continued practice and success, your new skills will become stronger and easier for you to put into practice. In this phase of treatment, we will ask you to begin to develop your WAIT skill and also to think about specific plans that will assist you as you move toward termination of your treatments and a continued recovery.

Watch	• Use the FEEL skill to get ready to WAIT. • Recovery is about being aware of yourself. • What are high-risk situations that you need to be aware of right now?
All	• What are your urges? • Are you at risk of other self-damaging behaviors in addition to eating disorder behaviors?
Impulses	Avoid urges to: • Follow strict eating rules • Skip meals • Binge • Use drugs or alcohol recklessly • Be perfectionistic • Relate to others or yourself recklessly
Today	• Is your recovery an important part of your life today? • What will distract you from your recovery today and how can you stay focused? • How will you stay committed to your recovery today?

Relapse Prevention

As you near the end of treatment, it is important to think about ways of continuing your progress and avoiding future problems. Many people who have struggled with binge eating struggle with symptoms after they finish treatment, even if they have been doing well for a number of months or even years. However, you can prevent future problems by planning now.

RELAPSE is actually a two-part process, starting first with a *LAPSE*. A lapse is a slip, a single event of problem eating. *LAPSES* are very common. Even if things are going well now, people who have had problems with binge eating in the past often experience lapses or slips, especially in the first few months after finishing treatment. Lapses do not have to turn into relapses. A *RELAPSE* refers to regular binge eating on an ongoing basis.

LAPSE

List some examples of a LAPSE:

1. Feeling out of control when eating
2. Skipping meals
3. Having urges to binge when upset

4. _____
5. _____
6. _____

One problem that causes a lapse to turn into relapse is how the person *thinks about* the lapse. Black-and-white thinking patterns can be especially risky when it comes to the process of relapse. Research has shown that if you think of a lapse as all or nothing, assume that you've failed, that all your progress is down the drain, and blame yourself for the lapse, you are more likely to have a full blown relapse. If, instead, you think of the lapse as a learning experience and an opportunity to use your coping skills to get back on track, you are likely to return to your healthy patterns. It is crucial to come up with some plans to cope with a lapse to prevent it from becoming a relapse.

What would a RELAPSE be like for you (including eating, behaviors, thoughts, interpersonal patterns, feelings)?

_____
_____
_____
_____
_____
_____
_____
_____
_____
_____

(continued)

RELAPSE

Sometimes people end up having relapses, even if they have worked hard to prevent them. This does not mean that you have "failed." If you have a relapse, it is important to act as quickly as possible to get back on track. Often, this will involve getting additional support and/or treatment.

If you had a relapse and started to binge-eat on a regular basis, what steps would you take?

1. _____

2. _____

3. _____

4. _____

5. _____

Lapse Plans

It is important to realize that there is a risk you will have a lapse during your recovery. How you cope with the situation makes a tremendous difference. We strongly encourage you to use the skills you have learned in your treatment to assist you in this regard. Below, we have listed each of your skills. Please write down a few words to indicate how you might use each of these skills in the event of a lapse. Remember, it is best to be prepared and cope effectively. Recovery can be a difficult process but is still attainable. The main goal is to prevent a lapse from turning into a relapse.

FEEL

_____

_____

_____

_____

_____

CARE

_____

_____

_____

_____

_____

ACT

_____

_____

_____

_____

_____

GOAL

_____

_____

_____

_____

_____

(continued)

SAID

_____

_____

_____

_____

REAL

_____

_____

_____

_____

SPA

_____

_____

_____

_____

WAIT

_____

_____

_____

_____

Be sure you review your plan with your therapist. This is a very important part of your treatment, particularly as you near the end of treatment. Your recovery will continue long after your treatment has ended.

Questions to Ask Yourself If You Have a Slip or a Lapse

1. How are my eating patterns? Have I been eating regular meals and snacks? Have I been skipping meals?

2. Should I start/continue written self-monitoring using my CARE form?

3. Should I resume or do more detailed meal planning?

4. Have I been trying to diet or restrict my food intake too strictly? Am I avoiding certain foods?

5. What was the trigger of the lapse? What can I do to change my environment or reaction to the trigger to prevent the slip from reoccurring?

6. What feelings am I having? How can I use my FEEL skill?

7. Do I need to make my focus on my appearance more positive?

8. Do I need to work on my perceptions of myself and my standards for myself? Are my standards or expectations of myself unrealistic?

9. How am I feeling about myself and others? What role did my feelings play in how and why the lapse occurred?

10. Am I focusing on my weight, shape, and eating to distract myself from other things that are upsetting? How can I address these issues more directly?

11. How are my relationships? Was it an interpersonal problem that triggered the slip? How can I deal with the situation?

12. What skills can I use to get back on track?

13. How is my relationship with myself? Is it self-protecting and self-accepting? How can I change self-criticism, self-control, and self-neglect patterns?

Toward a Healthy Lifestyle

To avoid a relapse, you need to be able to confront stressors, expected or unexpected, with increasing confidence. It is important to continue to practice the skills that you have developed. If there is a stressor that you can predict, such as returning to school, a friend's wedding, moving, and so forth, it will be important to anticipate what will be difficult, plan ahead, talk it out with a friend, and make sure your meals are eaten as scheduled.

Listed are some of the skills to continue to practice:

FEEL

CARE

ACT

GOAL

SAID

REAL

SPA

WAIT

It is also very important to have a support network established now that treatment is ending. This may include:

Family and friends.

Support systems and groups, volunteer work, etc.

Individual, couple, or group therapy.

Develop a Healthy Positive and Balanced Lifestyle

Improvements in your eating disorder behaviors mean less time spent binge eating, purging, and focusing on eating, shape, and weight—and more time available to you than you previously had. Part of relapse prevention is to develop a general idea of how you would like to allot that extra time each week. Are there activities you would like to spend more time doing? What is an optimal schedule for a healthy lifestyle for you? What could you do to make your daily life more fun and satisfying for you?

Healthy Lifestyle Plan

Hours per Week	Describe Activities
	Work/School
	Physical activity
	Time alone, meditation, relaxation, spirituality
	Recreation, hobbies, cultural pursuits
	Relationships
	Therapy/Support
	Meals (include grocery shopping and preparation of meals)
	Sleep

Finishing Treatment

As you finish treatment, you are probably having many thoughts and feelings. It is important to share these thoughts and feelings with your therapist. The end of treatment is a good time to review your progress and design a maintenance plan to continue your success.

What changes have you noticed since you started treatment in terms of . . .

Eating Patterns:

_____

_____

_____

How You Treat Yourself and Set Standards for Yourself:

_____

_____

_____

Behavior Patterns:

_____

_____

_____

Emotions and Feelings:

_____

_____

_____

Emotions and Feelings about Treatment Ending:

_____

_____

_____

Interpersonal Relationships:

_____

_____

_____

Other Changes:

_____

_____

_____

(continued)

After reviewing what you wrote on the previous page, think about what you can do to continue these changes. In writing your plan, pay close attention to things that have worked well for you during therapy that you can continue to do on an ongoing basis:

Plan

Eating Patterns:

_____

_____

_____

How You Treat Yourself and Set Standards for Yourself:

_____

_____

_____

Behavior Patterns:

_____

_____

_____

Emotions and Feelings:

_____

_____

_____

Interpersonal Relationships:

_____

_____

_____

Healthy Lifestyle:

_____

_____

_____

Other Strategies:

_____

_____

_____

Skill Cards

The FEEL Skill (Handout 5.5)

Focus	<ul><li>Find a quiet place.</li><li>Let yourself sit for a minute.</li><li>Pay attention to your body sensations.</li><li>Try not to judge or evaluate yourself.</li></ul>
Experience	<ul><li>Allow a feeling to come.</li><li>You may not know what to call it.</li><li>Pay attention to the feeling.</li><li>Practice staying with it for a while.</li><li>Notice how your body is feeling.</li></ul>
Examine	<ul><li>Start to wonder what this is.</li><li>What do you think this feeling is about?</li><li>Where is it coming from?</li></ul>
Label	<ul><li>Can you give it a name?</li><li>Try the name out. Does it fit?</li><li>Is that all of it, or is there another feeling? If yes, repeat.</li></ul>

The CARE Skill (Handout 6.2)

Calmly	<ul><li>Use the FEEL skill to get ready to CARE.</li><li>Find a quiet place that will help you remain calm.</li></ul>
Arrange	<ul><li>Work on your meal plan at least a day ahead of time.</li><li>Take time to plan what, when, and where you will eat.</li><li>Avoid eating anything that you haven't planned to eat.</li><li>Devote time each day to work on and follow your meal plan.</li></ul>
Regular	<ul><li>Eat regular meals and snacks to help prevent binge eating.</li><li>Try to get into a routine with your eating.</li><li>Follow your meal plan as closely as possible.</li></ul>
Eating	<ul><li>Understand that eating is an important part of self-care.</li><li>Check in with yourself about how you are feeling before, during, and after eating.</li><li>Try to allow yourself to eat a variety of food.</li><li>Experiment with eating differently.</li></ul>

The ACT Skill (Handout 6.7)

Adaptive	• Use the FEEL skill to get ready to ACT. • Can you identify your urge? • Can you identify your need? • Can you manage the urge and meet the need in a healthy way?
Coping	• Is there something you can do to solve the core problem? • Is this a situation that cannot be changed? • Can you change things if you wait? • Is it a time to self-soothe? • Is it a time to distract yourself? • Would your eating disorder behaviors really help?
Technique	• Coping is a skill that can be learned. • Coping efforts improve with practice. • What might help you to cope more effectively right now? • How can you meet your need differently?

The GOAL Skill (Handout 6.8)

Goals	• In 5 years, what do you hope will be true about your life? • Is the eating disorder part of your plan for the next 5 years? • What parts of your life do you want to develop or change in the next 5 years? • If you don't have goals, what interferes with setting some?
Objectives	• What goal are you working on today? • What will help you right now to reach your goal? • What could set you back in reaching your goal?
Affect	• If you reach your objective for today, how will you feel? What will it mean to you? • How can you manage urges today that could interfere with your objective?
Life-moments	• In this treatment we encourage you to try and change each moment. • This means trying to make choices and manage each situation you encounter without eating disorder behavior.

The SAID Skill (Handout 7.7)

Sensitively	• Use the FEEL skill before you speak (SAID). • Dealing with relationship problems is difficult, but it is part of your recovery. • Express your ideas, feelings, and needs respectfully. • Others might not change in response to your requests, but communicating with them is still valuable.
Assert	• You may want to "lay your cards on the table" honestly. • You may want to express an emotion, either positive or negative. • You may want to ask for something.
Ideas	• What is your opinion? • What do you believe? • What do you want? • What do you need?
Desires	• You may want to ask someone to do something for you. • You may want to express a desire to be closer to someone. • You may want to express a desire to separate from someone. • You may want to ask someone to do more or less of something.

The REAL Skill (Handout 7.10)

Realistic	• Use the FEEL skill to get ready to be REAL. • Being realistic means being fair and reasonable. • Draw conclusions based on the present moment, not the past.
Expectations	• Pay attention to the standards you set for yourself. • Are your goals fair and attainable? • If you don't reach a goal, can you credit yourself for trying? • Do the expectations you have for yourself reflect your values or somebody else's?
Affect	• Unrealistic self-standards and self-judgments can make you depressed, anxious, and frustrated. • What would it be like right now to be acceptable or good enough?
Living	• The way you evaluate yourself may affect your life goals. • The way you evaluate yourself may affect relationships. • Are you living your life with goals that you value?

The SPA Skill (Handout 7.14)

Self	• Use the FEEL skill to prepare for using the SPA skill. • Think about how you are relating to yourself. • Is the way that you are treating yourself in this moment healthy and adaptive?
Protect	• Recovery means protecting and caring for yourself. • Are you taking care of your needs, including food and eating? • How can you commit to your treatment and recovery as a way of caring for and protecting yourself?
Accept	• Are your goals fair and helpful? • What are you trying to accomplish? • How can you accept yourself and still strive for improvement? • How can you tolerate your limits or personal flaws? • Are there good things about yourself that you are currently ignoring?

The WAIT Skill (Handout 8.1)

Watch	• Use the FEEL skill to get ready to WAIT. • Recovery is about being aware of yourself. • What are high-risk situations that you need to be aware of now?	
All	• What are your urges? • Are you at risk of other self-damaging behaviors in addition to eating disorder behaviors?	
Impulses	Avoid urges to: • Follow strict eating rules • Binge • Be perfectionistic	• Skip meals • Use drugs or alcohol recklessly • Relate to others or yourself recklessly
Today	• Is your recovery an important part of your life today? • What will distract you from your recovery today and how can you stay focused? • How will you stay committed to your recovery today?	

References

Abdu, R. A., Garritano, D., & Culver, O. (1987). Acute gastric necrosis in anorexia nervosa and bulimia: Two case reports. *Archives of Surgery, 122*(7), 830–832.

Agras, W. S. (1991). Nonpharmacologic treatments of bulimia nervosa. *Journal of Clinical Psychiatry, 52,* 29–33.

Agras, W. S., Schneider, J. A., Arnow, B., Raeburn, S. D., & Telch, C. F. (1989). Cognitive-behavioral and response prevention treatments for bulimia nervosa. *Journal of Consulting and Clinical Psychology, 57,* 215–221.

Agras, W. S., Rossiter, E. M., Arnow, B., Schneider, J. A., Telch, C. F., Raeburn, S. D., et al. (1992). Pharmacologic and cognitive-behavioral treatment for bulimia nervosa: A controlled comparison. *American Journal of Psychiatry, 149,* 82–87.

Agras, W. S., & Telch, C. F. (1998). The effects of caloric deprivation and negative affect on binge eating in obese binge-eating disordered women. *Behavior Therapy, 29*(3), 491–503.

Agras, W. S., Walsh, T. B., Fairburn, C., Wilson, T., & Kraemer, H. C. (1999). A multicenter comparison of cognitive behaviour therapy and interpersonal psychotherapy in the treatment of bulimia nervosa. *Archive of General Psychiatry, 57,* 459–466.

Altabe, M., & Thompson, K. J. (1996). Body image: A cognitive self-schema construct. *Cognitive Therapy and Research, 20*(2), 171–193.

American Psychiatric Association. (1987). *Diagnostic and statistical manual of mental disorders* (3rd ed.). Washington, DC: Author.

American Psychiatric Association. (1994). *Diagnostic and statistical manual of mental disorders* (4th ed.). Washington, DC: Author.

American Psychiatric Association. (2013). *Diagnostic and statistical manual of mental disorders* (5th ed.). Arlington, VA: Author.

Ansell, E. B., Grilo, C. M., & White, M. A. (2012). Examining the interpersonal model of binge eating and loss of control over eating in women. *International Journal of Eating Disorders, 45*(1), 43–50.

Bardone-Cone, A. M., Wonderlich, S. A., Frost, R. O., Bulik, C. M., Mitchell, J. E., Uppala, S., et al. (2007). Perfectionism and eating disorders: Current status and future directions. *Clinical Psychology Review, 27*(3), 384–405.

Beck, A. T. (1967). *Depression: Clinical, experimental, and theoretical aspects.* New York: Harper & Row.

Beck, A. T. (1976). *Cognitive therapy and the emotional disorders.* New York: International Universities Press.

Beck, A. T. (1987). Cognitive models of depression. *Journal of Cognitive Psychotherapy, 1,* 5–37.

Benjamin, L. S. (1996). *Interpersonal diagnosis and treatment of personality disorders* (2nd ed.). New York: Guilford Press.

Benjamin, L. S. (2003). *Interpersonal reconstructive therapy: Promoting change in nonresponders.* New York: Guilford Press.

Berg, K. C., Crosby, R. D., Cao, L., Peterson, C. B., Engel, S. G., Mitchell, J. E, et al. (2013). Facets of negative affect prior to and following binge-only, purge-only, and binge/purge events in women with bulimia nervosa. *Journal of Abnormal Psychology, 122*(1), 111–118.

Berg, K. C., & Peterson, C. B. (2013). Assessment and diagnosis of eating disorders. In L. Choate (Ed.), *Eating and obesity: A counselor's guide to treatment and prevention* (pp. 91–118). Alexandria, VA: American Counseling Association.

Berkman, N. D., Lohr, K. N., & Bulik, C. (2007). Outcomes of eating disorders: A systematic review of the literature. *International Journal of Eating Disorders, 40*(4), 293–309.

Beutler, L., Malik, M., Alimohamed, S., Talebi, H., Noble, S., & Wong, E. (2004). Therapist variables. In Michael J. Lambert (Ed.), *Bergin and Garfield's handbook of psychotherapy and behavior change* (5th ed., pp. 227–306). New York: Wiley.

Birketvedt, G. S., Drivenes, E., Agledahl, I., Sundsfjord, J., Olstad, R., & Florholmen, J. R. (2006). Bulimia nervosa: A primary defect in the hypothalamic–pituitary–adrenal axis? *Appetite, 46*(2), 164–167.

Bordin, E. S. (1979). The generalizability of the psychoanalytic concept of the working alliance. *Psychotherapy: Theory, Research and Practice, 16*(3), 252–260.

Bornovalova, M. A., Gratz, K. L., Daughters, S. B., Nick, B., Delany-Brumsey, A., Lynch, T. R., et al. (2008). A multimodal assessment of the relationship between emotion dysregulation and borderline personality disorder among inner-city substance users in residential treatment. *Journal of Psychiatric Research, 42*(9), 717–726.

Bravender, T., & Story, L. (2007). Massive binge eating, gastric dilatation and unsuccessful purging in a young woman with bulimia nervosa. *Journal Adolescent Health, 41*(5), 516–518.

Brown, A., Mountford, V., & Waller, G. (2013). Therapeutic alliance and weight gain during cognitive behavioural therapy for anorexia nervosa. *Behaviour Research and Therapy, 51,* 216–220.

Brownell, K. D., Marlatt, G. A., Lichtenstein, E., & Wilson, G. T. (1986). Understanding and preventing relapse. *American Psychologist, 41,* 765–782.

Bruch, H. (1973). *Eating disorders: Obesity, anorexia nervosa, and the person within.* New York: Basic Books.

Bulik, C. M., Sullivan, P. F., & Epstein, L. H. (1992). Drug use in women with anorexia and bulimia nervosa. *International Journal of Eating Disorders, 11,* 213–225.

Burns, D. D., & Auerbach, A. (1996). Therapeutic empathy in cognitive-behavioral therapy: Does it really make a difference? In P. M. Salkovskis (Ed.), *Frontiers of cognitive therapy* (pp. 135–164). New York: Guilford Press.

Campos, J. J., Frankel, C. B., & Camras, L. (2004). On the nature of emotion regulation. *Child Development, 75*(2), 377–394.

Campos, J. J., Walle, E. A., Dahl, A., & Main, A. (2011). Reconceptualizing emotion regulation. *Emotion Review, 3*(1), 26–35.

Carney, C. P., & Andersen, A. E. (1996). Eating disorders guide to medical evaluation and complications. *Psychiatric Clinics of North America, 19*(4), 657–679.

Cassin, S. E., & von Ranson, K. M. (2005). Personality and eating disorders: A decade in review. *Clinical Psychology Review, 25*(7), 895–916.

Clarkin, J. F., & Levy, K. N. (2004). The influence of client variables in psychotherapy. In M. J. Lambert (Ed.), *Bergin and Garfield's handbook of psychotherapy and behavior change* (5th ed., pp. 194–226). New York: Wiley.

Constantino, M. J., Arnow, B. A., Blasey, C., & Agras, W. S. (2005). The association between patient characteristics and the therapeutic alliance in cognitive-behavioral and interpersonal therapy for bulimia nervosa. *Journal of Consulting and Clinical Psychology, 73*, 203–211.

Constantino, M. J., & Smith-Hansen, L. (2008). Patient interpersonal factors and the therapeutic alliance in two treatments for bulimia nervosa. *Psychotherapy Research, 18*(6), 683–698.

Cooper, P. J., & Fairburn, C. G. (1986). The depressive symptoms of bulimia nervosa. *British Journal of Psychiatry, 148*, 268–274.

Crosby, R. D., Wonderlich, S., Engel, S., Simonich, H., Smyth, J. M., & Mitchell, J. E. (2009). Daily mood patterns and bulimic behaviors in the natural environment. *Behaviour Research and Therapy, 47*, 181–188.

Crow, S. J., Agras, W. S., Halmi, K., Mitchell, J. E., & Kraemer, H. C. (2002). Full syndromal versus subthreshold anorexia nervosa, bulimia nervosa, and binge eating disorder: A multicenter study. *International Journal of Eating Disorders, 32*(3), 309–318.

Crow, S. J., Mitchell, J. E., Crosby, R. D., Swanson, S., Wonderlich, S. A., & Lancaster, K. (2009). The cost effectiveness of cognitive behavioral therapy for bulimia nervosa delivered via telemedicine versus face to face. *Behaviour Research and Therapy, 47*, 451–453.

Curry, S., Marlatt, G. A., & Gordon, J. R. (1987). Abstinence violation effect: Validation of an attributional construct with smoking cessation. *Journal of Consulting and Clinical Psychology, 55*, 145–149.

Cyders, M. A., & Smith, G. T. (2010). Longitudinal validation of the urgency traits over the first year of college. *Journal of Personality Assessment, 92*(1), 63–69.

D'Zurilla, T. J., & Goldfried, M. R. (1971). Problem solving and behavior modification. *Journal of Abnormal Psychology, 78*(1), 107–126.

Davis, R., Freeman, R. J., & Garner, D. M. (1988). A naturalistic investigation of eating behaviour in bulimia nervosa. *Journal of Consulting and Clinical Psychology, 56*, 273–279.

Ekman, P., & Friesen, W. V. (2003). *Unmasking the face: A guide to recognizing emotions from facial clues.* Los Altos, CA: Major Books.

Engel, S. G., Boseck, J. J., Crosby, R. D., Wonderlich, S. A., Mitchell, J. E., Smyth, J., et al. (2007). The relationship of momentary anger and impulsivity to bulimic behavior. *Behaviour Research and Therapy, 45*, 437–447.

Fairburn, C. G. (1997). Interpersonal psychotherapy for bulimia nervosa. In D. M. Garner & P. E. Garfinkel (Eds.), *Handbook of treatment for eating disorders* (2nd ed., pp. 278–294). New York: Guilford Press.

Fairburn, C. G. (2008). *Cognitive behavior therapy and eating disorders.* New York: Guilford Press.

Fairburn, C. G., & Harrison, P. J. (2003). Eating disorders. *Lancet, 351*, 407–416.

Fairburn, C. G., Jones, R., Peveler, R. C., Hope, R. A., & O'Connor, M. (1993a). Psychotherapy and bulimia nervosa: Longer-term effects of interpersonal psychotherapy, behavior therapy, and cognitive behavior therapy. *Archives of General Psychiatry, 50*, 419–428.

Fairburn C. G., Marcus, M. D., & Wilson, G. T. (1993b). Cognitive-behavioral therapy for binge eating and bulimia nervosa: A comprehensive treatment manual. In C. G. Fairburn & G. T. Wilson (Eds.), *Binge eating: Nature, assessment and treatment* (pp. 361–404). New York: Guilford Press.

Fairburn, C. G., Norman, P. A., Welch, S. L., O'Connor, M. E., Doll, H. A., & Peveler, R. C. (1995). A prospective study of outcome in bulimia nervosa and the long-term effects of three psychological treatments. *Archives of General Psychiatry, 52*, 304–312.

Fairburn, C. G., Welch, S. L., & Doll, H. (1997). Risk factors for bulimia nervosa: A community-based case-control study. *Archives of General Psychiatry, 54*, 509–517.

Farach, F. J., & Mennin, D. S. (2007). Emotion-based approaches to the anxiety disorders. In J. Rottenberg & S. L. Johnson (Eds.), *Emotion and psychopathology: Bridging affective and clinical science* (pp. 243–261). Washington, DC: American Psychological Association.

Feinstein, R. E., & Feinstein, M. S. (2004). Psychotherapy for health and lifestyle change. *Journal of Clinical Psychology, 57*, 1263–1275.

Ferrari, E., Magri, F., Pontiggia, B., Rondanelli, M., Fioravanti, M., Solerte, S. B., et al. (1997).

Circadian neuroendocrine functions in disorders of eating behavior. *Eating and Weight Disorders, 2*(4), 196–202.

Fichter, M. M., & Quadflieg, N. (2004). Twelve-year course and outcome of bulimia nervosa. *Psychological Medicine, 34*(8), 1395–1406.

Fischer, S., Peterson, C. M., & McCarthy, D. (2013). A prospective test of the influence of negative urgency and expectancies on binge eating and purging. *Psychology of Addictive Behaviors, 27*(1), 294–300.

Flückiger, C., Del Re, A. C., Wampold, B. E., Symonds, D., & Horvath, A. O. (2012). How central is the alliance in psychotherapy? A multilevel longitudinal meta-analysis. *Journal of Counseling Psychology, 59*(1), 10–17.

Fox, H., Axelrod, S., Paliwal, P., Sleeper, J., & Sinha, R. (2007). Difficulties in emotion regulation and impulse control during cocaine abstinence. *Drug and Alcohol Dependence, 89*, 298–301.

Fox, H., Hong, K., & Sinha, R. (2008). Difficulties in emotion regulation and impulse control in recently abstinent alcoholics compared with social drinkers. *Addictive Behaviors, 33*, 388–394.

Gilbert, P. (2009). *The compassionate mind.* London: Constable & Robinson.

Gilbert, P. (2010). *Compassion focused therapy: Distinctive features.* London: Routledge.

Goldschmidt, A. B., Peterson, C. B., Wonderlich, S. A., Crosby, R. D., Engel, S. G., Mitchell, J. E., et al. (2013). Trait-level and momentary correlates of bulimia nervosa with a history of anorexia nervosa. *International Journal of Eating Disorders, 46*, 140–146.

Goldschmidt, A. B., Wonderlich, S. A., Crosby, R. D., Engel, S. G., Lavender, J. M., Peterson, C. B., et al. (2014). Ecological momentary assessment of stressful events and negative affect in bulimia nervosa. *Journal of Consulting and Clinical Psychology, 82*(1), 30–39.

Goldstein, D. J., Wilson, M. G., Thompson, V. L., Potvin, J. H., & Rampay, A. H., Jr. (1995). Fluoxetine bulimia research group: Long-term fluoxetine treatment of bulimia nervosa. *British Journal of Psychiatry, 166*, 660–666.

Goss, K., & Allan, S. (2014). The development and application of compassion-focused therapy for eating disorders. *British Journal of Clinical Psychology, 53*, 62–77.

Gratz, K. L. (2007). Targeting emotion dysregulation in the treatment of self-injury. *Journal of Clinical Psychology, 63*(11), 1091–1103.

Gratz, K. L., & Roemer, L. (2004). Multidimensional assessment of emotion regulation and dysregulation: Development, factor structure, and initial validation of the difficulties in emotion regulation scale. *Journal of Psychopathology and Behavioral Assessment, 26*(1), 41–54.

Gratz, K. L., Rosenthal, M. Z., Tull, M. T., Lejuez, C. W., & Gunderson, J. G. (2006). An experimental investigation of emotion dysregulation in borderline personality disorder. *Journal of Abnormal Psychology, 115*(4), 850–855.

Gratz, K. L., & Tull, M. T. (2010). The relationship between emotion dysregulation and deliberate self-harm among inpatients with substance use disorders. *Cognitive Therapy and Research, 34*(6), 544–553.

Graybiel, A. M. (2008). Habits, rituals, and the evaluative brain. *Annual Review of Neuroscience, 31*, 359–387.

Greenfeld, D., Mickley, D., Quinlan, D. M., & Roloff, P. (1995). Hypokalemia in outpatients with eating disorders. *American Journal of Psychiatry, 152*(1), 60–63.

Grilo, C. M., Pagano, M. E., Skodol, A. E., Sanislow, C. A., McGlashan, T. H., Gunderson, J. G., et al. (2007). Natural course of bulimia nervosa and of eating disorder not otherwise specified: 5-year prospective study of remissions, relapses, and the effects of personality disorder psychopathology. *Journal of Clinical Psychiatry, 68*(5), 738–746.

Grilo, C. M., & Shiffman, S. (1994). Longitudinal investigation of the abstinence violation effect in binge eaters. *Journal of Consulting and Clinical Psychology, 62*, 611–619.

Gross, J. J. (1998). The emerging field of emotion regulation: An integrative review. *Review of General Psychology, 2*(3), 271–299.

Gross, J. J., & Feldman-Barrett, L. (2011). Emotion generation and emotion regulation: One or two depends on your point of view. *Emotion Review, 3*(1), 8–16.

Gyurak, A., Gross, J. J., & Etkin, A. (2011). Explicit and implicit emotion regulation: A dual-process framework. *Cognition and Emotion, 25*(3), 400–412.

Haedt-Matt, A. A., & Keel, P. K. (2011). Revisiting the affect regulation model of binge eating: A meta-analysis of studies using ecological momentary assessment. *Psychological Bulletin, 137*(4), 660–681.

Hatch, A., Madden, S., Kohn, M., Clarke, S., Touyz, S., & Williams, L. M. (2010). Anorexia nervosa: Towards an integrative neuroscience model. *European Eating Disorders Review, 18*(3), 165–179.

Haynos, A. F., & Fruzzetti, A. E. (2011). Anorexia nervosa as a disorder of emotion dysregulation: Evidence and treatment implications. *Clinical Psychology: Science and Practice, 18*(3), 183–202.

Heatherton, T. F., & Baumeister, R. F. (1991). Binge eating as escape from self awareness. *Psychological Bulletin, 110*, 86–108.

Herman, C. P., & Polivy, J. (1975). Anxiety, restraint, and eating behavior. *Journal of Abnormal Psychology, 84*(6), 66–72.

Herzog, D. B., Keller, M. B., Sachs, N. R., Yeh, C., & Lavori, P. W. (1992). Psychiatric comorbidity in treatment-seeking anorexics and bulimics. *Journal of the American Academy of Child and Adolescent Psychiatry, 31*, 810–818.

Higgins, E. T. (1987). Self-discrepancy: A theory relating self and affect. *Psychological Review, 94*, 319–340.

Hill, C. E., & Knox, S. (2009). Processing the therapeutic relationship. *Psychotherapy Research, 19*(1), 13–29.

Hoek, H. W. (2006). Incidence, prevalence and mortality of anorexia nervosa and other eating disorders. *Current Opinion in Psychiatry, 19*(4), 389–394.

Hoek, H. W., & van Hoeken, D. (2003). Review of the prevalence and incidence of eating disorders. *International Journal of Eating Disorders, 34*, 383–396.

Hohlstein, L. A., Smith, G. T., & Atlas, J. G. (1998). An application of expectancy theory to eating disorders: Development and validation of measures of eating and dieting expectancies. *Psychological Assessment, 10*(1), 49–58.

Holderness, C. C., Brooks-Gunn, J., & Warren, M. P. (1994). Co-morbidity of eating disorders and substance abuse review of the literature. *International Journal of Eating Disorders, 16*, 1–34.

Horvath, A. O. (2000). The therapeutic relationship: From transference to alliance. *Journal of Clinical Psychology, 56*(2), 163–173.

Hudson, J. I., Hiripi, E., Pope, H. G., Jr., & Kessler, R. C. (2007). The prevalence and correlates of eating disorders in the National Comorbidity Survey Replication. *Biological Psychiatry, 61*(3), 348–358.

Humphrey, L. L. (1986). Family dynamics in bulimia. *Adolescent Psychiatry: Developmental and Clinical Studies, 13*, 315–330.

Humphrey, L. L. (1987). A comparison of bulimic-anorexic and non-distressed families using structural analysis of social behavior. *Journal of the American Academy of Child and Adolescent Psychiatry, 26*, 248–255.

Humphrey, L. L. (1989). Observed family interactions among subtypes of eating disorders using structural analysis of social behavior. *Journal of Consulting and Clinical Psychology, 57*, 206–214.

Jimerson, D. C., Wolfe, B. E., Brotman, A. W., & Metzger, E. D. (1996). Medications in the treatment of eating disorders. *Psychiatric Clinics of North America, 19*, 739–754.

Johnson, C., & Larson, R. (1982). Bulimia: An analysis of moods and behavior. *Psychosomatic Medicine, 44*, 341–351.

Jones K. D., Burckhardt, C. S., & Bennett J. A. (2004). Motivational interviewing may encourage exercise in persons with fibromyalgia by enhancing self efficacy. *Arthritis and Rheumatism, 51*, 864–867.

Kappas, A. (2011). Emotion is not just an alarm bell—it's the whole tootin' fire truck. *Cognition and Emotion, 25*(5), 785–788.

Kaye, W. H., Weltzin, T. E., Hsu, L. K., McConaha, C. W., & Bolton, B. (1993). Amount of calories retained after binge eating and vomiting. *American Journal of Psychiatry, 150*(6), 969–971.

Keel, P., & Mitchell, J. E. (1997). Outcome in bulimia nervosa. *American Journal of Psychiatry, 154,* 313–321.

Keel, P. K., Mitchell, J. E., Miller, K. B., Davis, T. L., & Crow, S. J. (1999). Long-term outcome of bulimia nervosa. *Archives of General Psychiatry, 56*(1), 63–69.

Kelly, A. C., & Carter, J. C. (2014). Self-compassion training for binge eating disorder: A pilot randomized controlled trial. *Psychology and psychotherapy: Theory, research and practice* (pp. 1–19).

Kendler, K. S., MacLean, C., Neale, M., Kessler, R., Heath, A., & Eaves, L. (1991). The genetic epidemiology of bulimia nervosa. *American Journal of Psychiatry, 148,* 1627–1637.

Keys, A. Brožek, J., Henschel, A., Mickelsen, O., & Taylor, H. L. (1950). *The biology of human starvation* (2 vols.). Oxford, UK: University of Minnesota Press.

Kirchner, T. R., Shiffman, S., & Wileyto, E. P. (2012). Relapse dynamics during smoking cessation: Recurrent abstinence violation effects and lapse-relapse progression. *Journal of Abnormal Psychology, 121*(1), 187–197.

Laessle, R. G., Wittchen, H., Fichter, M. M., & Pirke, K. M. (1989). The significance of subgroups of bulimia and anorexia nervosa: Lifetime frequency of psychiatric disorders. *International Journal of Eating Disorders, 8,* 569–574.

Lambert, M. J. (Ed.). (2004). *Bergin and Garfield's handbook of psychotherapy and behavior change* (5th ed.). New York: Wiley.

Lavender, J. M., Wonderlich, S. A., Engel, S. G., Gordon, K., Kaye, W. H., & Mitchell, J. E. (2015). Dimensions of emotion dysregulation in anorexia nervosa and bulimia nervosa: A conceptual review of the empirical literature. *Clinical Psychology Review, 10,* 111–122.

Lewis, M., Haviland-Jones, J. M., & Barrett, L. F. (Eds.). (2008). *Handbook of emotions* (3rd ed.). New York: Guilford Press.

Loeb, K. L., Wilson, G. T., Labouvie, E., Pratt, E. M., Hayaki, J., Walsh, T. B., et al. (2005). Therapeutic alliance and treatment adherence in two interventions for bulimia nervosa: A study of process and outcome. *Journal of Consulting and Clinical Psychology, 73,* 1097–1107.

Maddocks, S. E., Kaplan, A. S., Woodside, D. B., Langdon, L., & Prian, N. (1992). Two-year follow-up of bulimia nervosa: The importance of abstinence as the criterion of outcome. *International Journal of Eating Disorders, 12*(2), 133–141.

Marlatt, G. A. (1996). Taxonomy of high-risk situations for alcohol relapse: Evolution and development of a cognitive-behavioral model. *Addiction, 91,* 37–49.

Marlatt, G. A., & Gordon, J. R. (Eds.). (1985). *Relapse prevention: Maintenance strategies in the treatment of addictive behaviors.* New York: Guilford Press.

Mennin, D. S., McLaughlin, K. A., & Flanagan, T. J. (2009). Emotion regulation deficits in generalized anxiety disorder, social anxiety disorder, and their co-occurrence. *Journal of Anxiety Disorders, 23*(7), 866–871.

Miller, W. R., & Rollnick, S. (1991). *Motivational interviewing: Preparing people to change addictive behavior.* New York: Guilford Press.

Miller, W. R., & Rollnick, S. (2002). *Motivational interviewing: Preparing people for change* (2nd ed.). New York: Guilford Press.

Miller W. R., & Rollnick, S. (2012). Meeting in the middle: Motivational interviewing and self-determination theory. *International Journal of Behavioral Nutrition and Physical Activity, 9,* 25.

Miller, W. R., & Sovereign, R. G. (1989). The check-up: A model for early intervention in addictive behaviors. In T. Loberg & W. R. Miller (Eds.), *Addictive behaviors: Prevention and early intervention* (pp. 219–231). Lisse, Netherlands: Swets & Zeitlinger.

Milos, G., Spindler, A., Ruggiero, G., Klaghofer, R., & Schnyder, U. (2002). Comorbidity of obsessive–compulsive disorders and duration of eating disorders. *International Journal of Eating Disorders, 31*(3), 284–289.

Mitchell, J. E., Agras, S., Crow, S., Halmi, K., Fairburn, C. G., Bryson, S., et al. (2011). Stepped care and cognitive-behavioural therapy for bulimia nervosa: Randomised trial. *British Journal of Psychiatry, 198*(5), 391–397.

Mitchell, J. E., & Crow, S. (2006). Medical complications of anorexia nervosa and bulimia nervosa. *Current Opinion in Psychiatry, 19*(4), 438–443.

Mitchell, J. E., Crow, S., Peterson, C. B., Wonderlich, S., & Crosby, R. (1998). Feeding laboratory studies in patients with eating disorders. *International Journal of Eating Disorders, 24*, 115–124.

Mitchell, J. E., Hatsukami, D., Eckert, E. D., & Pyle, R. L. (1985a). Characteristics of 275 patients with bulimia. *American Journal of Psychiatry, 4*, 482–485.

Mitchell, J. E., Davis, L., & Goff, G. (1985b). The process of relapse in patients with bulimia. *International Journal of Eating Disorders, 4*, 457–463.

Mitchell, J. E., Hatsukami, D., Pyle, R. L., & Eckert, E. D. (1986). The bulimia syndrome: Course of the illness and associated problems. *Comprehensive Psychiatry, 27*, 165–170.

Mitchell, J. E., Hatsukami, D., Pyle, R., & Eckert, E. D. (1988). Bulimia with and without a family history of drug abuse. *Addictive Behaviors, 13*, 245–251.

Mitchell, J. E., Hoberman, H. N., Peterson, C. B., Mussell, M., & Pyle, R. L. (1996). Research on the psychotherapy of bulimia nervosa: Half empty or half full. *International Journal of Eating Disorders, 20*, 219–229.

Mitchell, J. E., Pyle, R. L., & Eckert, E. D. (1991a). Sauna abuse as a clinical feature of bulimia nervosa. *Psychosomatics: Journal of Consultation Liaison Psychiatry, 32*, 417–419.

Mitchell, J. E., Pyle, R. L., Eckert, E. D., Hatsukami, D., Pomeroy, C., & Zimmerman, R. (1990). A comparison study of antidepressants and structured intensive group psychotherapy in the treatment of bulimia nervosa. *Archives of General Psychiatry, 47*, 149–157.

Mitchell, J. E., Pyle, R. L., & Hatsukami, D. (1991b). Enema abuse as a clinical feature of bulimia nervosa. *Psychosomatics: Journal of Consultation Liaison Psychiatry, 32*, 102–104.

Moyers, T. B., & Rollnick S. (2004). A motivational interviewing perspective on resistance in psychotherapy. *Journal of Clinical Psychology, 58*, 185–193.

Murphy, R., Straebler, S., Cooper, Z., & Fairburn, C. G. (2010). Cognitive behavioral therapy for eating disorders. *Psychiatric Clinics of North America, 33*(3), 611–627.

Mussell, M. P., Mitchell, J. E., Fenna, C. J., Crosby, R. D., Miller, J. P., & Hoberman, H. M. (1997). A comparison of onset of binge eating versus dieting in the development of bulimia nervosa. *International Journal of Obesity, 21*, 353–360.

Muehlenkamp, J. J., Engel, S. G., Wadeson, A., Crosby, R. D., Wonderlich, S. A., Simonich, H., et al. (2009). Emotional states preceding and following acts of non-suicidal self-injury in bulimia nervosa patients. *Behaviour Research and Therapy. 47*(1), 83–87.

National Institute for Clinical Excellence. (2004). *Eating disorders: Core interventions in the treatment and management of anorexia nervosa, bulimia nervosa, and related eating disorders* (NICE Clinical Guideline No. 9). London: Author.

Olmsted, M. P., Kaplan, A., & Rockert, W. (1994). Rate and prediction of relapse in bulimia nervosa. *American Journal of Psychiatry, 151*, 738–743.

Pearson, C. M., Combs, J. L., Zapolski, T. C. B., & Smith, G. T. (2012). A longitudinal transactional risk model for early eating disorder onset. *Journal of Abnormal Psychology, 121*(3), 707–718.

Pearson, C. M., Wonderlich, S. A., & Smith, G. T. (in press). A risk and maintenance model for bulimia nervosa: From impulsive action to compulsive behavior. *Psychological Review.*

Peterson, C. B. (2005). Conducting the diagnostic interview. In J. E. Mitchell & C. B. Peterson (Eds.), *Assessment of eating disorders* (pp.32–58). New York: Guilford Press.

Powers, P. S. (1996). Initial assessment and early treatment options for anorexia nervosa and bulimia nervosa. *Psychiatric Clinics of North America, 19*, 639–655.

Roemer, L., Lee, J. K., Salters-Pedneault, K., Erisman, S. M., Orsillo, S. M., & Mennin, D. S. (2009). Mindfulness and emotion regulation difficulties in generalized anxiety disorder: Preliminary evidence for independent and overlapping contributions. *Behavior Therapy, 40*(2), 142–154.

Rossiter, E. M., Agras, W. S., Telch, C. F., & Schneider, J. A. (1993). Cluster B personality disorder characteristics predict outcome in the treatment of bulimia nervosa. *International Journal of Eating Disorders, 13*, 349–357.

Rottenberg, J., & Johnson, S. L. (2007). *Emotion and psychopathology: Bridging affective and clinical science*. Washington, DC: American Psychological Association.

Ruderman, A. J., Belzer, L. J., & Halperin, A. (1985). Restraint, anticipated consumption, and overeating. *Journal of Abnormal Psychology, 94*(4), 547–555.

Ruderman, A. J., & Grace, P. S. (1987). Bulimics and restrained eaters: A personality comparison. *Addictive Behaviors, 13*, 359–368.

Russell, G. (1979). Bulimia nervosa: An ominous variant of anorexia nervosa. *Psychological Medicine, 9*, 429–488.

Safer, D. L., Telch, C. F., & Agras, W. S. (2001). Dialectical behavior therapy for bulimia nervosa. *American Journal of Psychiatry, 158*(4), 632–634.

Safer, D. L., Telch, C. F., & Chen, E. Y. (2009). *Dialectical behavior therapy for binge eating and bulimia*. New York: Guilford Press.

Safran, J. D., & Muran, J. C. (2000). Resolving therapeutic alliance ruptures: Diversity and integration. *Journal of Clinical Psychology, 56*(2), 233–243.

Safran, J. D., Muran, J. C., & Eubanks-Carter, C. (2011). Repairing alliance ruptures. *Psychotherapy, 48*(1), 80–87.

Safran, J. D., Muran, J. C., & Samstag, L. W. (2002). Repairing alliance ruptures. In J. C. Norcross (Ed.), *Psychotherapy relationships that work: Therapist contributions and responsiveness to patients* (pp. 235–254). London: Oxford University Press.

Safran, J. D., & Segal, Z. V. (1996). *Interpersonal process in cognitive therapy*. Northvale, NJ: Jason Aronson.

Selby, E. A., Anestis, M. D., & Joiner, T. E. (2008). Understanding the relationship between emotional and behavioral dysregulation: Emotional cascades. *Behaviour Research and Therapy, 46*(5), 593–611.

Simmons, M. S., Grayden, S. K., & Mitchell, J. E. (1986). The need for psychiatric-dental liaison in the treatment of bulimia. *American Journal of Psychiatry, 143*, 783–784.

Smith, G. T., Simmons, J. R., Flory, K., Annus, A. M., & Hill, K. K. (2007). Thinness and eating expectancies predict subsequent binge-eating and purging behavior among adolescent girls. *Journal of Abnormal Psychology, 116*(1), 188–197.

Smyth, J., Wonderlich, S. A., Heron, K., Sliwinski, M., Crosby, R. D., Mitchell, J. E., et al. (2007). Daily and momentary mood and stress predict binge eating and vomiting in bulimia nervosa patients in the natural environment. *Journal of Consulting and Clinical Psychology, 75*, 629–638.

Smyth, J. M., Wonderlich, S. A., Sliwinski, M. J., Crosby, R. D., Engel, S., Mitchell, J. E., et al. (2009). Ecological momentary assessment of affect, stress, and binge-purge behaviors: Day of week and time of day effects in the natural environment. *International Journal of Eating Disorders, 42*, 429–436.

Stice, E. (2001). A prospective test of the dual pathway model of bulimic pathology: Mediating effects of dieting and negative affect. *Journal of Abnormal Psychology, 110*, 124–135.

Stice, E. (2002). Risk and maintenance factors for eating pathology: A meta-analytic review. *Psychological Bulletin, 128*, 825–848.

Stice, E., & Agras, W. W. (1998). Predicting the onset and remission of bulimic behaviors in adolescence: A longitudinal grouping analysis. *Behavior Therapy, 29*, 257–276.

Stice, E., Schupak-Neuberg, E., Shaw, H. E., & Stein, R. I. (1994). Relation of media exposure to eating disorder symptomatology: An examination of mediating mechanisms. *Journal of Abnormal Psychology, 103*, 836–840.

Strauman, T. J. (1989a). Self-discrepancies in clinical depression and social phobia: Cognitive structures that underlie emotional disorders? *Journal of Abnormal Psychology, 98*, 5–14.

Strauman, T. J. (1989b). The paradox of the self: Psychodynamic/social-cognitive integration. In R. C. Curtis (Ed.), *Self-defeating behaviors: Experimental findings, clinical impressions, and practical implications* (pp. 311–339). New York: Plenum Press.

Strauman, T. J., & Glenberg, A. M. (1994). Self-concept and body-image disturbance: Which self-beliefs predict body size overestimation? *Cognitive Therapy and Research, 18*, 105–125.

Strauman, T. J., Vookles, J., Berenstein, V., Chaiken, S., & Higgins, E. T. (1991). Self-discrepancies and vulnerability to body dissatisfaction and disordered eating. *Journal of Personality and Social Psychology, 61*, 946–956.

Striegel-Moore, R. H., Silberstein, L. R., & Rodin, J. (1986). Toward an understanding of risk factors for bulimia. *American Psychologist, 41*, 246–263.

Strober, M., & Humphrey, L. L. (1987). Familial contributions to the etiology and course of anorexia nervosa and bulimia. *Journal of Consulting and Clinical Psychology, 55*, 654–659.

Strober, M., & Katz, J. L. (1988). Depression in the eating disorders: A review and analysis of descriptive, family and biological findings. In D. M. Garner & P. E. Garfinkel (Eds.), *Diagnostic issues in anorexia nervosa and bulimia nervosa* (pp. 80–111). New York: Brunner/Mazel.

Thomas, J. J., Crosby, R. D., Wonderlich, S. A., Striegel-Moore, R. H., & Becker, A. E. (2011). A latent profile analysis of the typology of bulimic symptoms in an indigenous Pacific population: Evidence of cross-cultural variation in phenomenology. *Psychological Medicine, 41*(1), 195–206.

Thomas, J. J., Vartanian, L. R., & Brownell, K. D., (2009). The relationship between eating disorder not otherwise specified (EDNOS) and officially recognized eating disorders: Meta-analysis and implications for DSM. *Psychological Bulletin, 135*(3), 407–433.

Thompson, R. A. (1994). Emotion regulation: A theme in search of definition. *Monographs of the Society for Research in Child Development, 59*(2–3), 25–52.

Thompson, J. K., Heinberg, L. J., Altabe, M. N., & Tantleff-Dunn, S. (1999). *Exacting beauty: Theory, assessment and treatment of body image disturbance.* Washington, DC: American Psychological Association.

Treasure, J. L., Katzman, M., Schmidt, U., Troop, N., Todd, G., & de Silva, P. (1999). Engagement and outcome in the treatment of bulimia nervosa: First phase of a sequential design comparing motivation enhancement therapy and cognitive behavioural therapy. *Behaviour Research and Therapy, 37*, 405–418.

Verplanken, B., & Orbell, S., (2003). Reflections on past behavior: A self-report index of habit strength. *Journal of Applied Social Psychology, 33*, 1313–1330.

Vieth, A. Z., Strauman, T. J., Kolden, G. G., Woods, T. E., Michels, J. L., & Klein, M. H. (2003). Self-System Therapy (SST): A theory-based psychotherapy for depression. *Clinical Psychology: Science and Practice, 10*, 245–268.

Vitousek, K., Watson, S., & Wilson, G. T. (1998). Enhancing motivation for change in treatment resistant eating disorders. *Clinical Psychology Review, 18*, 391–420.

Walsh, B. T., (2013). The enigmatic persistence of anorexia nervosa. *American Journal of Psychiatry, 170*, 477–484.

Walsh, B. T., Kissileff, H. R., & Hadigan, C. M. (1989). Eating behavior in bulimia. In L. H. Schneider & S. Cooper (Eds.), *Psychobiology of human eating disorders: Preclinical and clinical perspectives* (pp. 446–455). New York: New York Academy of Sciences.

Watkins, E. R., & Nolen-Hoeksema, S., (2014). A habit-goal framework of depressive rumination. *Journal of Abnormal Psychology, 123*, 24–34.

Welch, S. L., & Fairburn, C. G. (1996). Impulsivity or comorbidity in bulimia nervosa: A controlled study of deliberate self-harm and alcohol and drug misuse in a community sample. *British Journal of Psychiatry, 169*, 451–458.

Wildes, J. E., & Marcus, M. D. (2011). Development of emotion acceptance behavior therapy for anorexia nervosa: A case series. *International Journal of Eating Disorders, 44*(5), 421–427.

Wildes, J. E., Ringham, R. M., & Marcus, M. D. (2010). Emotion avoidance in patients with anorexia nervosa: Initial test of a functional model. *International Journal of Eating Disorders, 43*(5), 398–404.

Williams, A. D., & Grisham, J. R. (2012). Impulsivity, emotion regulation, and mindful attentional focus in compulsive buying. *Cognitive Therapy and Research, 36*(5), 451–457.

Williams, A. D., Grisham, J. R., Erskine, A., & Cassedy, E. (2012). Deficits in emotion regulation associated with pathological gambling. *British Journal of Clinical Psychology, 51*(2), 223–238.

Wilson, G. T., Fairburn, C., Agras, W. S., Walsh, B. T., & Kraemer, H. (2002). Cognitive-behavioral therapy for bulimia nervosa: Time course and mechanisms of change. *Journal of Consulting and Clinical Psychology, 70*(2), 267–274.

Wilson, G. T., Grilo, C. M., & Vitousek, K. M. (2007). Psychological treatment of eating disorders. *American Psychologist, 62*(3), 199–216.

Wilson, G. T., & Zandberg, L. J. (2012). Cognitive-behavioral guided self-help for eating disorders: Effectiveness and scalability. *Clinical Psychology Review, 32*(4), 343–357.

Wood, W., & Neal, D. T., (2007). A new look at habits and the habit-goal interface. *Psychological Bulletin, 114*, 843–863.

Woods, D. W., Himle, M. B., & Conelea, C. A., (2006). Behavior therapy: Other interventions for tic disorders. *Advances in Neurology, 99*, 234–240.

Wonderlich, S. A. (1992). Relationship of family and personality factors in bulimia nervosa. In J. H. Crowther, D. L. Tannenbaum, S. E. Hobfoll, & M. A. P. Stephens (Eds.), *The etiology of bulimia nervosa: The individual and familial context* (pp. 170–196). Washington, DC: Hemisphere.

Wonderlich, S. A., Brewerton, T., Jocic, Z., Dansky, B., & Abbott, D. W. (1997). The relationship between childhood sexual abuse and eating disorders. *Journal of the American Academy of Child and Adolescent Psychiatry, 36*, 1107–1115.

Wonderlich, S. A., de Zwaan, M., Mitchell, J. E., Peterson, C., & Crow, S. (2003). Psychological and dietary treatments of binge eating disorder: Conceptual implications. *International Journal of Eating Disorders, 34*, 558–573.

Wonderlich, S. A., Engel, S. G., Peterson, C. B., Robinson, M. D., Crosby, R. D., Mitchell, J. E., et al. (2008). Examining the conceptual model for integrative cognitive-affective therapy for BN: Two assessment-related studies. *International Journal of Eating Disorders, 41*, 748–754.

Wonderlich, S. A., Klein, M. H., & Council, J. R. (1996). Relationship of social perceptions and self-concept in bulimia nervosa. *Journal of Consulting and Clinical Psychology, 64*(6), 1231–1237.

Wonderlich, S. A., & Mitchell, J. E. (1997). Eating disorders and comorbidity: Empirical, conceptual, and clinical implications. *Psychopharmacology Bulletin, 33*, 3981–3901.

Wonderlich, S. A., Peterson, C. B., Crosby, R. D., Smith, T. L., Klein, M. H., Mitchell, J. E., et al. (2014). A randomized controlled comparison of integrative cognitive-affective therapy (ICAT) and cognitive-behavioral therapy-enhanced (CBT-E) for bulimia nervosa. *Psychological Medicine, 44*(3), 543–553.

Index

Note: Page numbers in *italics* indicate figures and tables.